PRAISE

for Cherie Kephart and
A Few Minor Adjustments

"With raw guts, wisdom, and a spirit as tenacious as they come, Cherie tells the story of her harrowing experience with an undiagnosed condition in a way that will keep you wanting to turn the page. Intelligent, tender, and triumphant, *A Few Minor Adjustments* is a must read."

—Marni Freedman, editor, and award-winning author
of *Playing Mona Lisa* and *7 Essential Writing Tools*

"*A Few Minor Adjustments* is everything you want in a book. I was drawn in from the first sentence and pulled quickly to the last beautiful sentence. It is magnificent, reflective, truly touching, and meaningful, with the welcomed relief of the perfect touch of humor condensing twenty years of life with the right amount of detail for one to grasp and feel part of her story—and it is a great story!"

—Dr. Melinda Nevins, D.O.

"Cherie ⬝⬝⬝⬝⬝⬝⬝⬝⬝⬝⬝⬝⬝⬝⬝⬝⬝⬝⬝⬝⬝⬝⬝⬝⬝⬝⬝⬝⬝⬝⬝⬝ ersonal, her
vulneral ⬝⬝⬝⬝⬝⬝⬝⬝⬝⬝⬝⬝⬝⬝⬝⬝⬝⬝⬝⬝⬝⬝⬝⬝⬝ make this a
universa ⬝⬝⬝⬝⬝⬝⬝⬝⬝⬝⬝⬝⬝⬝⬝⬝⬝⬝⬝⬝⬝⬝⬝⬝⬝⬝

First Reads

"Cherie Kephart's *A Few Minor Adjustments* takes you on a perilous inner and outer journey to places and dangers into an unknown that even the most seasoned adventurer would fear to tread, and in doing so teaches us by courageous example how to survive by the only available resources we have when all else is lost; wit, humor, and perseverance."

—Matthew J. Pallamary, author of
Spirit Matters and *Land Without Evil*

"Cherie brings a delicate balance of humor and brutal honesty to a tale that would be dark and grim in the hands of a lesser writer. That she is here to even tell her story is a miracle—that she has the talent and insight to tell it so brilliantly is a gift for us all."

—Jeff Thurman, author and retired FBI agent

"A powerful, gripping, and insightful story that keeps you engaged and wanting to read more. Reading someone else's brutally honest struggle makes you thankful for what you have—and what you don't have! Cherie Kephart is a living tribute to learning how to laugh at life and see the light and lesson in every dire situation."

—Dr. Kevin Grold, Ph.D. in psychology
and CEO at EDReferral.com

"Cherie's will to persevere, in spite of ongoing disappointment and daunting circumstances, holds up a beacon of hope for others who may be dealing with similar difficulties."

—Beverly Hamowitz, licensed clinical social worker

"With *A Few Minor Adjustments*, Cherie Kephart communicates an important message to the many people struggling with undiagnosed illnesses and their friends and relatives, who want to help them, but don't know how—you are not alone. The struggle is real and prevalent. This story not only shares Ms. Kephart's experiences, from her time in Africa to the mounting health issues she faced back home, but it starts an important conversation about our society and how we handle health problems that are not clearly defined."

—Lindsey Salatka, author of *Fish Heads and Duck Skin*

"*A Few Minor Adjustments* is the moving, heartwarming memoir of Cherie's courageous struggle and eventual triumph and is sure to inspire others who suffer with never-ending pain."

—Roger L. Conlee, author of *Dare the Devil*,
The Hindenburg Letter, and other historical novels

"Everyone has been physically ill at one point or another, and it's rarely pleasant. Cherie's treatment of such a difficult, personal topic is nothing short of lovely. It's a story celebrating life. We all need that, even when we're healthy."

—Reina Menasche, social worker and
author of *Silent Bird* and *Twice Begun*

"Cherie's fighting spirit and ability to keep moving forward when one answer means dozens of new questions is both inspiring and nourishing to anyone who faces a similar experience in the medical world or in any aspect of life."

—Asa Wild, mother of three beautiful children,
one who had an extremely rare metabolic disorder

"In today's world of social media, hand-held devices, work, and family responsibilities, infrequently do I pick up a good book, but after I picked up *A Few Minor Adjustments*, I could not put it down. Cherie Kephart's memoir is filled with adventure, heroes, villains, and beautiful descriptions. Most outstanding is her sense of humor that carried her through her medical challenges. As a physician and cancer survivor, I appreciate her strength and perseverance that others facing known and unknown diseases will be inspired by."

—Dr. Sharon Sternfeld, MD, FAAP, Dr. Good-for-children

"After her excruciating ordeal, Cherie has re-opened her heart to write this vivid account of her courageous journey, leaving readers with an inspiring message and a sense of awe."

—Peggy Lang, editor, ghostwriter, and co-author
of the award winning novel, *Assassin's Game*

A FEW MINOR ADJUSTMENTS

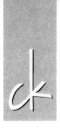

A FEW MINOR ADJUSTMENTS

a memoir of healing

CHERIE KEPHART

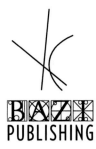

BAZI
PUBLISHING

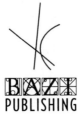

PUBLISHING

Bazi Publishing
San Diego, CA
BaziPublishing.com

For more information, email bazi@bazipublishing.com
or visit BaziPublishing.com

PUBLISHER'S CATALOGING-IN-PUBLICATION DATA

Names: Kephart, Cherie, author.

Title: A few minor adjustments : a memoir of healing / Cherie Kephart.

Description: San Diego, CA : Bazi Publishing, [2017]

Identifiers: ISBN: 978-1-947127-00-5 (hardback) | 978-1-947127-01-2 (paperback) | 978-1-947127-02-9 (epub) | 978-1-947127-05-0 (audio book) | LCCN: 2017905877

Subjects: LCSH: Kephart, Cherie--Health. | Chronically ill--Biography. | Chronic diseases--Diagnosis. | Healing--Psychological aspects. | Patients' writings.| LCGFT: Autobiographies. | BISAC: BIOGRAPHY & AUTOBIOGRAPHY / Personal Memoirs. | BIOGRAPHY & AUTOBIOGRAPHY / Medical. | BODY, MIND & SPIRIT / Inspiration & Personal Growth. | BODY, MIND & SPIRIT / Healing / General. | HEALTH & FITNESS / Diseases / General.

Classification: LCC: RC108 .K46 2017 | DDC: 362.1/092--dc23

Printed in the United States of America
10 9 8 7 6 5 4 3 2 1

Book Jacket and Page Design: Asa Wild
Elephant Artwork provided by: Getty Images
Author's Photograph: Brigid Parsons

For Alex

AUTHOR'S NOTES

This is a true story. At least the way I remember it.

Most of the names and any distinguishing characteristics of the persons included in this book have been changed to protect their privacy.

If you learn anything from this book and decide to abruptly change your life, it is not my fault. But any laughter you experience, I'll take credit for that.

"If you're going through hell, keep going."

—Winston Churchill

chapter one

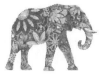

ENTERING
THE UNKNOWN

APRIL 2004, PART I – SAN DIEGO

Hard water hit my breasts. The musty odor of old pipes filled my nostrils. I coughed and turned in circles in my shower, observing the cracked tiles beneath my feet, stepping carefully around them because I had been cut before. I avoided the large patches of mold covering the rusty handles and walls. No matter how much I scrubbed, this cottage was run-down and full of spores.

Damn landlord never fixes a thing.

I lathered my skin with soap, breathing in the scent of citrus as I scoured the crevices that had collected sand from playing beach volley-ball earlier that evening. The image of Alex entered my mind; his short brown hair, crystal-blue eyes, full ruby lips, and olive skin. I envisioned his tall, lean, and muscular body pressing up against me as we made love. I had only known him for a few months, but we were enamored with one another. We met while I was working as a technical writer at a software company. We became friends, sharing our adoration for animals, love for exercise, thirst for intellectual conversation, and desire to spend quiet time in nature. My thirty-third birthday was in a few weeks and I wondered what we would do to celebrate.

I turned to rinse the soap from my back and felt a sharp biting pain in my neck. I dropped to the hard tile floor. Water pounded over my head. I tried to stand, to move my neck, but the pain intensified like a saw ripping my flesh and muscles apart. I screamed.

I crawled out of the shower and across the floor.

Focus. Get to the phone. Call for help.

I inched across the living room floor, one arm limp by my side, the other forcing me along like an oar wading through sand. I reached the phone and dialed.

Pick up. Please.

"Hello?"

"Alex?" My voice felt shallow. My wet hand gripped the receiver.

"Cherie. You all right?"

"No." I strained to speak. "Intense pain. I collapsed." I forced words into the air between breaths. "My neck feels—broken. I don't know how, but I can't feel my left arm. I'm scared, Alex."

"Hang on, CK, I'll come right over."

I dropped the phone. I had suffered chronic throbbing neck pain for years from a car accident when I was twenty-one, but this felt as if a lion had ripped apart my neck with its teeth. I inched from the kitchen back to the bathroom. Heard the water still running from the shower. I pushed along the rough hardwood floor. Long, sopping hair covered my face.

My concentration weakened. Heat radiated from my neck into my limbs. My legs burned.

Just get to the bathroom.

My arms and legs quivered. I pushed myself up using both sides of the door jamb. I entered the cramped, steamy shower. Turned the handle enough to halt most of the flowing water. The shower head continued to drip, but I didn't care.

I groaned, forcing myself down the corridor to my bedroom. Holding my neck with my right hand, I climbed wet and naked onto the mattress. My neck stiffened as if my muscles were filled with cement. From the corner of my eye I saw my digital alarm clock on the nightstand, but the numbers looked hazy: 8, 4, 5. 8:45 p.m. The drive from Alex's studio apartment would be at least thirty minutes. Would I make it that long?

Goose bumps prickled across my arms and legs. I wrapped myself in a golden throw that hung over the edge of the bed. The dampness of my skin made me tremble. I swayed back and forth in tiny movements and started to cry.

A tidal wave of tension rushed through me. I grimaced and turned toward the clock. 8:52. *Please hurry, Alex* echoed in my head like a mantra.

I thought back to my visit to the hospital two weeks earlier. The ER smelled like bleach and fear. Fluorescent lights shone brightly overhead. I sat on a gurney in a busy hallway and watched the flurry of activity. My knee ached and my heart pounded like an elephant stampeding after too much Red Bull and cocaine. Something was wrong with me and I trusted that the medical system would agree and offer me an efficient way to heal.

A red-haired doctor with bushy eyebrows rushed up to me. "What did you find?" I asked him.

He paused, shaking his head. "Your EKG's a bit, well, unusual," said Dr. Unsure, as I had come to think of him.

Just say it, I can take it.

"It's your heart. Your EKG readings are reversed." He fiddled with his stethoscope.

"What's that mean?"

"I'm not sure," said Dr. Unsure. "Very unusual." He scratched his head, thought for a moment. "I've never seen this before, but I don't believe there's anything to worry about right now."

So, the time to worry would be when?

"I need you to do a follow-up with your primary doctor, a cardiologist, and a neurologist. You seem stable enough for now."

Stable enough?

I drove home with fifty less dollars in my checking account and a thousand more worries.

Sharp stinging sensations crept up my neck to the base of my head, bringing me back to the moment. Still in my cottage. 9:01. My hands shook as I propped myself up. The wet blanket fell to the floor. I stumbled toward my closet, panting as I shoved clothes aside with my right arm, searching for a loose T-shirt and sweatpants. I situated the shirt around my neck and torso; the cotton fabric stuck to my damp breasts. I struggled, pulling down the shirt, still crying, still shaking.

I bent over to lift my sweatpants, fumbled with my left leg, then dropped my right leg gingerly into the hole, and finally pulled the pants up around my waist.

Shoes. Easy shoes. I slid my feet into my sandy flip flops.

What else? ID. Insurance card. Purse.

I turned toward the hallway, and a bolt of pain sledgehammered my neck. I grabbed my head and fell to the floor.

Red numbers glowed out of the corner of my eye. 9:15. The clock mocked me. I dragged myself toward the living room. My purse dangled on the edge of a chair. I stretched out toward the bag, grabbed it, and crumpled onto the carpet. I tried to inhale but could only produce curt, shallow breaths.

Please, someone help me!

I heard a car door slam. Harnessing strength, I pushed myself up from the floor and limped to the door.

Alex's voice sounded muffled through the thick wooden door. "Cherie. Open up."

I wanted to scream out to him, but my voice was a breathless rasp. I cried as I unlocked and pulled the door open.

Alex towered over me. His luminous blue eyes sparkled between his thick eyelashes, and a hazy white cloud highlighted his body. He looked like a savior. He stretched out his arms and gently wrapped them around me. I shook and sobbed. "What happened?" he asked.

"I don't know."

"I've got you, CK. Hang on." He lifted me into his arms and carried me to the car.

In the waiting room, Alex held me close and consoled me. The masculine aroma of perspiration and shampoo filled my nostrils as I nestled in his arms. I could feel the compassion in his touch. A serious man, Alex was a software engineer who had worked his way up to vice-president of a Fortune 500 company. A self-proclaimed "unforgiving bastard," but I had come to know his softer side. He often spent weekends volunteering at animal shelters, rescuing stray cats and finding them homes.

The emergency room bustled with activity. Nurses scurried from one side of the waiting area to the other. I surveyed the people around me and noticed a faint scent of blood. A disheveled, burly man with a stab wound sat alone staring at the floor, holding a blood-soaked wash cloth on the side of his stomach. Was it a bar fight, gang related, or some form of fatal attraction?

A quiet middle-aged Hispanic couple sat across from me. I couldn't discern the reason for their visit to the ER, or which one of them was sick. They watched me periodically, perhaps wondering what pathogen I had, and what, if anything, I infected their air with.

Was I contagious?

Alex kept his eyes on me, occasionally running his hand along my back or across my leg. His presence kept me sane.

We sat for hours in our awkward plastic waiting-room chairs. I focused on wanting to live, yet the pangs radiating from my neck and head raged as if a savage battle were being fought over my every muscle, sinew, and bone.

"Why's it taking so long? I can't stand this anymore."

"I know. This is awful. I'll ask the nurse again. You've got to hang on, CK."

Although Alex sat next to me, I somehow felt alone. He knew about the two other times I'd endured pain so overpowering that, unlike this day when I fought to live, I asked to die.

My heart rate accelerated as I recalled those times of despair and what I had survived. Did those two episodes give me the strength to overcome this new trial, or had they depleted my reservoir of endurance? Had they contributed to my current unknown condition?

I didn't know.

chapter two

PIONEERING
FOR PEACE

JANUARY 1994 – ZAMBIA

I was twenty-three years old the first time I wished for death. I was serving as a Peace Corps volunteer in Zambia. Twelve of us became the first group of volunteers. We would learn to speak the Bantu language, Bemba. We called ourselves the *Kalapashi*, meaning "the pioneers."

Before traveling to Africa, I absorbed the Peace Corps medical spokesperson's lecture on a multitude of precautions, preventive measures, consequences, and statistics. She described several diseases, emergencies, injuries, and accidents we were bound to encounter throughout our two-year service.

Each year millions of people around the world were infected with malaria. Between one and three million people died from this parasitic infection. Ninety percent of these deaths occurred in Africa. Besides the high risk of contracting malaria, HIV was prevalent. Statistics showed that approximately eighty-five percent of Peace Corps volunteers had sexual relations while in their host country. Heterosexual transmission of HIV in the United States represented eight percent. In Africa, it was eighty percent. There were thirteen million cases of HIV in the world. Eight million of those were in Africa. Fifty percent of hospital patients there had HIV. Hospitals and medical clinics commonly reused needles for immunizations and blood drawing because supplies were low. Instead of sterilizing, they washed the needles in hot water.

Aside from warning us about venomous snakes, crocodiles, and spiders, they warned us about dysentery, giardia, hepatitis, and a wide variety of water-borne diseases like schistosomiasis. Equipped with all of this staggering information, I assured myself that for the duration of my service I would always boil and treat my drinking water (even before brushing my teeth), consistently take my prophylactic medications, sleep in a chemically treated mosquito net, stay current on my immunizations, abstain from sex, keep out of hospitals and medical clinics, and avoid swimming in any body of water.

Being young, unhampered, and idealistic, I decided I would remain healthy by adhering to the rules and guidelines and remain conscious of everything I did. My young mind propelled me forward without fear. I joined the Peace Corps because I aspired to make my life mean something. I needed to believe I was imperishable. I kept thinking of a quote from Margaret Mead: "Never doubt that a group of thoughtful, committed citizens can change the world. Indeed, it's the only thing that ever has."

I wanted to be a part of that change. Never did I imagine that most of the change would be within me.

My first three months, from January to April, were with my eleven fellow volunteers in the south of Zambia, participating in language, technical, and cultural training. Each of us lived with a host family. Since Zambia had been a British colony, many of the locals in the larger cities spoke English. At the end of our three-month training we would be relocated to remote villages where almost only Bemba would be spoken.

During our training, we lived in Kabwe, an old zinc and lead mining town. Home to 200,000 residents, it offered few amenities. The middle of town had a large marketplace where hundreds of local vendors sold their agricultural and homemade goods. It smelled like charcoal and dust, surrounded by a steady stream of flies constantly circling and landing on the makeshift tables, food, and people. The training site, where we studied and gathered for Peace Corps events, was on the outskirts.

We were trained to orchestrate water and sanitation/health education projects; to build wells and latrines; and to educate the locals about good health practices to prevent disease. When I arrived, people bathed in, drank out of, urinated, and defecated near and in the same slow moving river that ran through the village. The degree of illness and death from contaminated water sources was alarming. Combined with deaths from malaria, HIV, and other causes, the average life expectancy of Zambians was around thirty-two years.

Despite my cautious intentions, illness managed to find me in interesting ways. In addition to changes in diet, such as fried caterpillars that tasted similar to burnt French fries, and newly found bowel functions that all of the volunteers enjoyed, I noticed three red sores, one on the inside of my right arm and two on my behind. At first they looked like pimples, so I ignored them, but after a few weeks, they grew bigger, darker red, and became so piercing it was difficult to sit.

The Peace Corps medical staff, a doctor and nurse who were both in Zambia for the first time, brought me into a small unused dorm room on the Peace Corps training campus to investigate the sores. The room smelled musty, had cold concrete floors and one window that was painted shut.

"Cherie, lie down on that cot and we'll take a look at you," Dr. Enthusiasm said, pointing to a child-sized mattress in the corner. He was a brown-haired Jerry Garcia look-a-like from Alabama. I wondered if he had ever been to a Grateful Dead concert. The nurse, a petite and naturally beautiful dark-haired woman from Alaska, smiled at me.

I positioned myself on the bed, lying backside up, and lowered my pants and underwear so they could see the two bright red sores on my butt. The two medical professionals rubbed, poked, and picked at the sores, chatting back and forth while I kept from fidgeting.

"We aren't certain, but we think you've contracted a Putzi fly or Tumbu fly infection. This is exciting." The doctor's voice cracked. "I've never seen it before, but I just read about it. It's native to Africa. The flies lay eggs in damp clothes hanging outside to dry. Once the clothes come into contact with human skin, the eggs hatch. The larvae burrow into the skin and, if left untreated, morph into adult maggots."

"Whoa. Did you say maggots?"

"Yes, maggots."

The muscles in my stomach tightened. "I have maggots in my butt?"

"It's been a few weeks since you first noticed them, correct?"

"Yes. But, oh gosh, how do we get them out?"

"We'll have to cut them out. It may be a little painful. You'll have to remain quite still, all right?"

I reached my arms up to grasp the thin metal frame of the bed. I shut my eyes. "Okay."

While the doctor rubbed the areas with a cold, wet antiseptic wipe, I braced myself. They used an X-Acto blade and a pair of tweezers, medical instruments resembling those included with the board game Operation.

The sharp blade cut into my flesh. Lying face down, I couldn't see what they were doing with these elementary tools, but it sounded like an archaeological investigation being conducted on my butt cheeks.

"That's interesting. Wait, I have it. Nope, I lost it. Wait, I have it. No, it burrowed back in again. We've got to cut a little more. Okay, now dig." Their less than comforting dialogue, coupled with their probing and cutting, continued for almost forty-five minutes, during which I thought so many things. What was I doing here? Maybe I made a mistake? Who was I kidding? Get these things out of me! Was I strong enough for this? Was I prepared? How does one prepare for getting maggots in her butt? I knew that the Peace Corps experience was not for the weak hearted, but I didn't know it was going to be this tough. I was not in a hospital or a medical clinic (which I wanted to avoid, so how could I complain?), but in a random, non-sterile room with no pain medication in sight. Just me, two perplexed medical staff with tools from their portable first-aid kit, and three determined worms.

"We've got it!" they exclaimed when they finally extracted the first maggot from my aching ass. "Do you want to see it?"

I was not in the mood for show and tell. But they showed me a cream-colored worm about a half an inch long wriggling on the end of the tweezers before I had a chance to respond. It looked about as happy as I did.

"Do you need to take a break or should we continue?"

My glute muscles ached as if they had been stung by a swarm of wasps. "No break, let's get the other two out of me." I closed my eyes and waited for the cold, sharp blade to once again cut into the fatty flesh on my behind.

The second one didn't take as long, perhaps ten minutes total.

"Not too much blood. That wasn't bad," they said to me with mild excitement.

My butt cheeks didn't agree, but with only one worm left in my body, I felt relieved. After they cleaned the areas and placed bandages on the two holes, I pulled up my underwear and pants and turned onto my side so they could address the last worm in my arm. I felt nauseated and fidgeted.

The nurse held my arm as the doctor picked at my flesh with the small, shiny blade. "Okay, hold still."

"I'm trying."

"Sorry, Cherie, not you, the worm."

"Oh."

"I have it," Dr. Enthusiasm said. "Oh no. That's not good."

I looked at my bicep where the freeloading worm vacationed, but the nurse and doctor hovered over me, and I couldn't see what they were doing. "What happened?"

"Ah. I grabbed a hold of it, but I think it broke in half. See?" The lifeless half worm sprinkled in blood drooped on the tweezers.

"Where's the other half?"

The nurse swallowed and with a sheepish expression said, "I think it went back in your arm."

Having half of a worm inside me felt worse than having the whole thing. What if it couldn't be retrieved? What would happen then?

I felt beads of sweat form on my back. I wanted Dorothy's ruby slippers to click me back to the time before maggots invaded my flesh. After more excavating and tweezing, the other half of the worm eventually came out of my arm.

The next day, the nurse explained that she had researched further into Putzi fly infections.

"It turns out they are easily prevented and treated," the nurse said with a proud voice. "To prevent them, you must iron all of your clothes. The heat kills the eggs and stops them from making their way into your skin. To remove a worm, spread Vaseline on the infected area. It cuts off the air supply to the maggot. In order not to suffocate, it comes out on its own."

"Wait. If we had simply spread a dollop of Vaseline on my skin, the maggots would have come out on their own?"

"It seems so. Well, at least now we know." The nurse sported a half grin.

Just call me Guinea, last name Pig.

My encounter with these little scrounging creatures prevented others from suffering the same fate. John, one of my fellow volunteers, was a twenty-three-year-old New Yorker who was deaf since a young age, had wavy brown hair, clear-rimmed glasses and hearing aids, and always wore long pants, long-sleeved shirts, and sweatshirts with hoods. He often removed his hearing aids, covered his head with his hood, and tuned out the world.

John's words came soft, lower than a whisper. "Cherie, what did the nurse say?"

I mouthed, "Iron all clothes."

He looked confused. "Really?"

"Yup. Another item to add to the must-do list." I giggled.

He smiled and gave me a warm, comforting hug.

It was a lesson I only needed to learn once, but without electricity, this was not an easy task. After hand-washing and line-drying my clothes, I used a coal iron over each article, including socks, bras, underwear, and even shoelaces. Laundry day became an all-day event, but it was worth the effort. My clothes looked nicely pressed, and more importantly, I was maggot-free.

By April, I had completed my three-month training and felt ready to apply what I had learned. Eager to help improve the water and waste management of the villagers I had yet to meet, my impassioned enthusiasm clouded the details of what lay ahead. I didn't envision living in an isolated village, not knowing anyone, digging wells and latrines in the hot African sun surrounded by disease and death. I envisioned hope, friendship, peace, and health.

chapter three

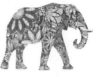

LIVING THE DREAM

APRIL 1994 – ZAMBIA

My new place in the world would be a little village in northern Zambia called Mulundu. I pledged to help however I could.

Mulundu, located in an area called Luapula, sat between the main road and the Luapula River, which flowed from north to south. This river, the main water source for the entire province, was warm from the sun, contaminated with disease, and inhabited by crocodiles. Less than twenty miles west of it was politically unstable Zaire. The Peace Corps told me not to go there under any circumstances. Another thing to add to the do-not-do list.

I began wondering what it was I *could* do here.

Numerous mud-brick huts with thatched roofs lined the village and spread out amongst miles of open land. Row after row, anemic brown color and similar shapes blended together with the dry landscape. Tall, barren bushes lined the vicinity of the village. Sparse trees with wide-arching branches grew throughout the area, most prominently by the river.

There were no modern amenities. No paved roads, grocery stores, post offices, telephones, restaurants, hospitals, or shops of any kind. People had barely enough food to feed themselves.

The majority of the villagers had no private transportation. Most of them ventured no farther than they could travel by foot. The only public transportation was an unreliable bus system that ran along the main dirt road and had no schedules. If I wanted to catch one of the rundown buses, I had to wait, usually for hours. Often night came and I had to try again the next day. Although the Peace Corps discouraged us from doing so, I came to learn that hitchhiking was the easiest way to travel.

I lived in a thatched-roof mud hut with a family of three while a brick house was being built for me. I was told the construction could take at least four to six months depending on supplies and the availability of labor, so I remained living with my host family, the Chipilis.

Agnes, the wife and mother, was in her late twenties. She had toffee-colored skin, a broad nose, a long neck, and short dark hair always hidden beneath an indigo-and-coral scarf wrapped around her head. The husband and father, Fewdays Chipili, had recently turned thirty, yet had the innocent eyes of a child. His skin looked at least five shades darker than Agnes's. His full black beard and mustache contrasted with his bright white teeth. Their son, Cadbury, was only two. He had a smooth complexion, wide, deep brown eyes, and pouty lips. Weeks before he was born, the Chipilis were given a gift from a British missionary passing through the village: a small box of Cadbury chocolates. This was the first time either of them had ever tasted chocolate. They were so impressed by the delicious and unique flavor they named their only child after the gift.

Fewdays was a slender man, five-feet-ten inches tall and only one-hundred-and-twenty pounds. His father, the eldest of the living Chipilis, called Ba Chipili (Ba is a sign of respect), was in his late fifties. One evening over dinner, he told me the story of how he had given his son that name.

"My son was born almost dead," Ba Chipili said in Bemba. "We saw he wouldn't live long. Maybe a few days. So, why not give him that name?" His mouth opened wide into a toothless smile. "But he lived. The name reminds us to give thanks he is still here."

It was not uncommon for several children in a family to die before the age of five from disease or malnourishment. Fewdays was the sixth child in their family, and only the second to survive.

The first time I met the Chipilis, I tumbled out of the Peace Corps Land Cruiser and saw Fewdays grinning, his eyes wide open. He stood tall in front of his modest mud hut with his hands clasped together. Agnes huddled next to him, holding Cadbury in her arms. Agnes smiled only slightly, exhibiting her bashfulness. Cadbury stared straight at me, watching my every move. He never smiled. This was the first time he had ever seen a white person.

Less than ten minutes after my arrival, my two duffel bags of belongings were inside the mud hut, and the Peace Corps vehicle maneuvered down the decrepit road kicking up auburn dust in its tracks.

Upon entering the hut with the Chipilis for the first time, I panicked.

A little voice inside my head said: *Crap. This is real. This is the next two years of my life.* I swallowed hard and ignored the uneasiness building in my chest. *You wanted adventure. Well, you've got it.*

I didn't yet know just how right that little voice would be.

Fewdays, Agnes, and Cadbury all slept in one room on an old mattress covered with a cotton sheet and frayed, thick gray blanket, all of which rested on a dirt floor. I slept in the other room on a similar mattress on the same dirt floor, with similar bedding covered by a large white mosquito net I had bought in Kabwe. The doors to the two bedrooms were made of splintered wood that did not reach the ceiling or floor. The third room in the house served as an entryway. It had three rickety wooden chairs and a square table. There was no kitchen, bathroom, or any other rooms. The toilet was something for me to build, outside, and the kitchen was a cleared dirt area with coals in the ground behind the hut.

With no electricity, or running water, I ate what they ate, and slept when and how they slept—except for my mosquito repellent and netting. Mr. Chipili, as I called him at first, was the only one who could speak English and cheerfully helped me practice speaking Bemba.

On my first solo trek around the village, I waved at women working with crops and caring for their children as they cooked and swept around their huts. Some children played in the dirt, ran, laughed, and smiled. They had no toys, only sticks and rocks, but their imaginations were intact. One group of kids used a stick as a cricket bat and a rock as the ball. A few kids even built small structures as if they were using Legos. I noticed other children sitting on rocks, near the edge of the river, their emaciated bodies circled by flies, their eyes sunken, some even missing limbs. A few men gathered in an open area and drank the locally brewed beer.

As I searched for possible sites to build a communal latrine, I noticed much more than I ever thought I would see. The people of Mulundu had deep, dark skin that glistened in the sunlight. They were slender yet muscular from hauling water from the river, and growing crops such as millet. Most walked barefoot, adorned by tattered and worn clothes, but some wore old suits, sports T-shirts, or old 1970s style floral blouses donated from overseas charities. One man wore a complete 1980s navy-blue McDonald's uniform, equipped with matching hat and belt. He walked proud in his polyester garb, strutting through the center of the village, even in 110 degree heat. I doubted he was lost for work. The nearest McDonald's restaurant was at least a full-day drive and an airplane ride away.

When I walked closer to the outskirts of the village, I noticed illness more. Several children had malnourished bodies, untreated lesions, and protruding stomachs swollen from disease. Their eyes appeared weary, their bodies folded over in limp, almost lifeless positions. When they saw me, they stared and smiled, and for a moment I could see resilience in their eyes.

A cascade of new sights, sounds, and scents flooded me. Varied voices speaking Bemba, long stretches of inhospitable landscape, and the bitter aroma of the locally fermented alcohol mixed with the smell of burning charcoal. Taken aback by the people and the magnitude of suffering, I soon became absorbed in self-doubt. Could I possibly make any difference?

I thought I was prepared to live alone in this unfamiliar and secluded place, but the isolation and distant way of life felt overwhelming. A few thousand people lived in the village of Mulundu, yet the remoteness of this strange place induced loneliness. My upbringing near the beach in Southern California felt like a dream. I believed living in the United States was a privilege. But experiencing this contrast felt heavy.

As I made my way back to the other side of the village toward my hut, a bell clanged. I tracked the sound and stumbled upon a church, located in the south end of the village. The beauty of the bell gave me hope that indeed serenity existed somewhere in Mulundu.

At dinner that evening, I told Fewdays about my first trek around the village.

"I am so glad you are finding your way around. Now, please eat, Miss Cherie." Fewdays motioned to the food in the center of the table.

"Thank you." I reached for a handful of *ubwali*, the local staple of boiled millet. I rolled it backward and forward in my palm, shaping the warm blob into a ball, a motion I copied from the locals back in Kabwe. They used it as a utensil to scoop up the rest of the food. I didn't know it then, but we would eat *ubwali* at every meal for the remainder of my stay. It tasted bland, and felt soft and comforting in a funny sort of way.

"Fewdays, I want to ask you, earlier today I saw a church...."

"Oh yes. We go. Maybe sometime you will join us?"

"That would be nice. So, I heard the bell ring. Was there church service today?"

"No, Miss Cherie, not today. Only on Sundays."

"Then why was it ringing?"

"We use the bell to alert the villagers when someone has died. It is our way of communicating, but also, respecting the dead."

My heart skipped. "Who died?"

"A man from the east part of the village was attacked by a crocodile down by the river. May he rest in peace."

"I'm so sorry, Fewdays. Did you know him?"

"Yes." Fewdays bowed his head. "A good man."

After that night, the bell no longer sounded beautiful and inviting; its noise felt haunting.

It rang almost every day.

I was not innocent enough to believe that death was not a part of life, but in my new African home, the ending of life was much more prevalent, much more inevitable. Death still evoked sadness and bereavement, but it was not unusual.

Even though I had only met a handful of people besides the Chipilis, many recognized me. Since there were no other non-Africans in the area, news journeyed fast about the blue-eyed blonde, young Caucasian woman from the United States living in Mulundu. A phenomenon the Peace Corps calls "the fishbowl effect." Many Zambians, especially children, stared, snickered, and followed me for long periods of time without uttering a word.

One day, a group of four children followed me on my early morning walk. They never spoke to me, they only giggled and pointed.

"Hello and good morning," I said, as we walked through the village. They stayed silent, surprised that I spoke Bemba.

With a smile I said, "How are you today?"

When I turned around and stepped forward, they whispered among themselves, covering their mouths with their hands.

They followed me through the narrow pathways around the village and back to my hut, waiting outside as I changed and prepared to bathe using a plastic bucket, a rag, and a bar of soap. I expected them to be gone when I came back out, but they were patient.

I prepared my sponge bath, which I took only two to three times a week because of the difficulty hauling water from the river. The children watched as I lifted a large plastic bucket filled with water over to a four-foot area surrounded by a flimsy wall of thatch that Fewdays and I had assembled to protect my privacy. Inside my open-air bath, I set down my soap, sponge, and towel. I needed to pee before bathing.

I walked out into the bush, hoping the children would realize I was going to relieve myself, but these children were curious and never strayed more than ten feet away from me. I had no choice, so I squatted behind an area of tall brush. The kids placed their hands on their faces only half covering their eyes and laughed.

All four children ambled behind me back to the bath area and loitered outside while I bathed. Once clean and dressed, I emptied the water and cleaned the area. I smiled at the children, but they only ogled me as if I was some type of white-skinned alien.

Day turned into night, and the children returned to their homes. They had spent the entire day watching me plod through my mundane daily tasks, such as ironing clothes and writing in my journal. As I helped Agnes prepare dinner that night, I asked her about the children in my limited Bemba.

"Did you see those children following me today?"

"Yes, Miss Cherie." Agnes continued to stir the millet with her brawny yet graceful arms.

"Why did they do that?"

Her voice came soft. Her bright smile and kind disposition matched her husband's. "They like you."

"They do? They didn't talk to me."

She glanced down at Cadbury, playing in the dirt next to us. "They like you, but are scared of you too."

I remembered the first time I met Cadbury. He stared at me from in between his mother's arms. I thought he was a bashful boy, but perhaps he was just shy around me.

"Why?"

"You are different."

"How can I get them to talk with me?"

Agnes paused, unsure of what I meant. Fewdays walked up behind me, hearing my question, "Patience is a virtue. They will get to know you, as we are. They need time."

I learned to expect these activities, to smile, and continue doing what I needed, but I stood out in a crowd. Once while traveling through a neighboring village, I met a man who knew of me, yet I did not know him.

"Miss, will you be so kind to deliver a message to my friend in Mulundu?" He nodded his head as if to answer for me.

"Okay, but my Bemba is very, ah, small." I didn't know the word for limited.

"Tell her that her brother told me the child to Cynthia is dead," he said without much expression.

Whoa. "Did you say Cynthia's child is dead?"

"Yes. Please tell her."

"I'm so sorry."

"Yes. So you deliver the message?"

"Maybe it would be better if you wrote it down." I pretended to scribble something.

"Please, deliver the message, yes?"

"I will."

After the man departed, I realized I did not even know the child's name. It took me hours of deliberation to decide how I would convey this grim news, and what of my limited Bemba vocabulary would soften what I needed to say. The woman I gave the message to was bereaved, but not surprised. She asked no questions of me, she just cried.

No matter how much illness and death surrounded me in Zambia, I viewed the passing of a human being as neither prosaic nor expected. Each time I attended a funeral, witnessed a loved one mourn, heard the bell in my village echo, or looked upon the eyes of a mother caring for her fragile and ailing child, I felt overwhelmed with a trembling fury of emotions, from anger, depression, shock, and denial, to a towering sense of compassion and duty. Unwilling to look away, I longed to live up to my ideals: to help those in need.

Even though I was young, resilient, and healthy, I was not naive enough to believe I could cure diseases and stop the multitude of deaths from bombarding these people, but I did believe I could stay healthy and make a small difference, if not in my entire village, at least in a few individuals' lives. I trusted that would be enough to keep me motivated for the next two years.

I was wrong.

It was a typical night in my village, "typical" meaning nothing much happened in Mulundu at night. Most activities occurred during the daytime, and I never strayed far away from my mud hut after dark since only the stars and the moon illuminated this secluded area.

The Chipilis and I ate pumpkin leaf, okra, and millet for dinner, the same food I had almost every day. Once we finished our food and our conversations ceased, the Chipilis headed off to their room, and I sought refuge underneath my mosquito netting with my journal, a tattered copy of Tolstoy's *War and Peace*, a red flashlight, and a half bottle of warm, boiled, iodine-treated water.

As I switched between reading and writing in my journal, I scratched at my arms, neck, and legs. My skin looked like inflamed Swiss cheese from the hundreds of mosquitoes which had been feasting on me. To no avail, I used special mosquito repellents, coils, candles, and netting. I wore long-sleeved shirts, pants, and thick socks, even when it was 110 degrees in a place without fans, much less air conditioning. The persistent flies were also annoying. They circled until I tired of waving my hands, and then landed once again to do whatever they do besides transport disease.

Thumbing through the pages of my book, I heard something in the thatch roof above me move. I shined my flashlight up and saw nothing, so I tricked myself into believing it was my old friends, whom I called Fred and Ethel.

During my time in Kabwe, my host family had provided me with a cozy room in their house, much bigger than my room in Mulundu. This room came equipped with one cot, one sheet, one blanket, one pillow, one cupboard to place my belongings in, and two sizable spiders, seemingly mounted on the ceiling. They were brown, with eight long, skeletal legs, and bulbous abdomens the size and shape of an apricot pit.

I never saw them move. Each night before I went to sleep, I checked that they were in their normal location. In the morning, I looked again to make certain they had stayed where I determined they should, in the farthest corner away from my bed. The family told me they were good to have in my room as they killed most other insects. I was instructed not to bother them. Disturbing them was the last thing I intended.

Although I am not arachnophobic, I did not want spiders as roommates, particularly ones that dwarfed baby rodents, but I decided if I had to live with them, I would give them names, so I called one Fred and the other Ethel.

I chose to believe that Fred and Ethel had somehow made the long trip north from Kabwe to join me in my village and had taken up residence in my new roof, watching over me while awaiting their next prey. That was the only way I would ever get any sleep.

Because I was focused on the clattery thatch above me, it took a while to notice the subtle sounds my stomach made. Soon, I could concentrate on nothing except my body, as I became lightheaded, nauseated, and dizzy. Without warning, I had what many of the volunteers called "The Big D." Having diarrhea is uncomfortable enough with a clean, private toilet, an abundance of double-ply toilet paper, an exhaust fan, a potent air freshener, soap, a large hand towel, and a sink with ample running water. All I had was a smelly hole in the ground located between a large rock and a scrawny shrub.

The Peace Corps did provide us with toilet paper, one rudimentary difference in the way I lived and the locals' lifestyle, which included neither toilet paper nor eating utensils. They used their left hands to wipe themselves and their right hands to eat. As one would expect, it was insulting to eat with or shake hands with the left hand. Being left-handed and not knowing this piece of useful information, I had obtained one of my first cultural lessons by reaching into the common serving dish with my left hand for some millet. Everyone stopped eating and gave me disapproving stares. Someone finally communicated that I had ruined dinner and offended the entire gathering. Following that incident, I sat on my left hand during mealtimes so I would not make that mistake twice.

Toilet paper could only be purchased in a few of the larger towns a couple of hours away, so I learned to ration it. With the forceful diarrhea I had that night, rationing it became impossible. Making it to my funky-smelling, fly-infested hole in the ground was my only priority.

Clutching my stomach, I climbed out from under my mosquito net, remembering to bring my flashlight and my trusty roll of rough toilet paper. I shook my hiking boots upside down to ensure no insects had crawled into them, slipped them on, and walked into the darkness and to the hole. The silence in that area impressed me. The Chipilis and all of the neighbors could hear every sound I made. I grunted and groaned only in my head as I made my way out into the bush, hoping to avoid any black mambas—one of Africa's most dangerous and feared snakes.

Months prior, back in Kabwe, I had almost run into a mamba— literally. While jogging early one morning, a long, fierce-looking snake slithered a few paces in front of me on the narrow dirt road. A nearby watchman for the local training facility leaped forward and cut it in half with his machete. He told me I should not be running in the morning, since it is the time when the snakes come out. Enough said. I never ran in the morning on that road again.

Thankfully, I found my way safely to the squalid hole. Once I finished, I staggered back to my hut, removed my boots, crawled back into my netting and collapsed on my mattress. Not more than three minutes passed before nature ordered me back out to the bush once again.

I repeated this routine for at least four hours. Sometimes I lasted thirty minutes between trips, and other times only five. I was running out of toilet paper, and my quadriceps ached. I became dehydrated. I had to keep my fluid intake up but I only had eight ounces of water to last me through the night. I planned to fetch some the following day and boil and treat it since my supply was low, but clean drinking water, or any water for that matter, was not easy to come by.

The main water source was the filthy river inhabited by crocodiles that can grow up to sixteen feet in length and weigh up to twenty-five hundred pounds. They sunbathe to aid their digestion and have at least two sets of teeth. Within the first month in my village, two locals were killed by them. I had every intention of limiting my time near the river to avoid disease as well as these human-eating animals. Unfortunately, I learned that crocodiles also travel up to a few miles on land, primarily at night. I hoped they weren't traveling near my hole. Most nights I tried to hold my bodily functions until daybreak, but on this night, there was no holding of anything.

On each of my treks out into the bush, I gripped the toilet paper, protecting it like gold. Although coarse, it was better than nothing at all and reminded me of something one of the other volunteers used to say, "Give me toilet paper or die!" I came to believe this as a valid threat, something I could see myself saying one day, if needed.

As the night progressed, I was faced with the likelihood that what remained of the puny roll would not be enough to sustain me through the rest of the night.

Back in my hut, underneath my mosquito net, I whispered into the night, "Please, make this stop."

I began to hallucinate, seeing black spiders the size of gorillas wearing bibs and drooling blood as they lunged at my neck. I squirmed and cowered underneath my blanket. I could no longer muster the energy to get outside, or even out of my room. I swallowed a packet of orange Gatorade powder, thirsted for a glass of ice-cold water, then blacked out.

The next morning, after repeated knocks on my door, Fewdays peered inside and found me half dressed, passed out on my mattress. A pile of clothes covered with spots of dried blood and a puddle of diarrhea sat next to me.

By coincidence or serendipity, another Peace Corps volunteer visited me that same day. When he found out what had happened, he hitched a ride to the nearest town and contacted the Peace Corps office. The next morning, I was medevacked to Lusaka, the capital of Zambia. The Peace Corps version of a medical evacuation included a three-hour ride in a dilapidated pickup truck filled with chickens, dodging herds of goats, a five-hour wait at the local air strip, and a turbulent ride in a rickety plane.

I recalled mumbling to Fewdays about the moving thatch ceiling in my room. He told me not to worry, and reassured me it was just some bats. He mentioned he had seen them before and would get rid of them before I returned.

Instead of spiders, I had bats. But if Fewdays said he was going to take care of something, he would, so I didn't worry about the bats. I was worried about what would happen to me. Dysentery could be fatal if not treated. I did not want to die—at least not yet, but that day was getting closer.

I arrived in southern Zambia, at the Lusaka airport. I was greeted by a driver named Boniface who wore a dirt-colored outfit and by a nurse named Delia sporting short, mousy brown hair and a pale complexion that mirrored her white shorts. She pushed a haggard assembly of rusted metal and torn cloth named Mr. Wheelchair. I was delighted to see them all.

chapter four

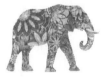

CLOSE ENCOUNTERS
OF THE CURIOUS KIND

APRIL 1994 – ZAMBIA

I woke to the distant sound of Delia singing along to the song *Africa* by Toto on her record player. She entered the guest room, stopped singing, and placed a plate of fried eggs, mango slices, and a glass of water on a tray next to me on the bed. "How you feeling this morning, Cherie?"

"A little better, thanks." My abdomen felt taut, my mouth parched. I sat up and reached for the glass.

Delia watched as I drank the water like a race car driver at a pit stop. An American nurse, wife, and devoted mother of three, she worked for the U.S. Embassy in Lusaka and part-time for the Peace Corps. "You've had a rough few days."

"Yeah, I suppose." Tiny pools of saliva formed in my mouth as I surveyed the food.

I took my first bite. My taste buds danced.

Delia watched me devour my breakfast. "I spoke with the Peace Corps Country Director this morning and—"

"Kyle?" I said with a mouth full of juicy mango.

She pushed a few strands of hair behind her ear, "Yeah, Kyle. He's arranged for one of the Peace Corps drivers to take you back to your village."

I stopped chewing. "I just got here yesterday."

"I know."

29

"Don't you think it's a bit soon?"

"It's hard to say since we're not sure what's wrong with you." She took my empty glass.

"Yesterday you said I have some kind of parasite or amoeba. Or giardia."

She placed a full glass on my tray. "All of your tests came back inconclusive. Parasites are difficult to detect. The two antibiotics you're taking are quite strong, especially Flagyl. They should kill whatever these bugs are. It may take a little time for you to regain your strength. I'll tell Kyle to postpone your return for a day or two so you can rest a little more."

I nodded, finished the last of my food, and thanked Delia for the delicious meal. I pushed the tray aside, pulled the sheets over me and slept another eight hours.

Two days later, though still shaky, I felt ready to return to Mulundu.

"Remember to finish all of the antibiotics and keep hydrated," Delia shouted as I waved from the slow-moving Peace Corps Land Cruiser.

"I will. Thank you again!" I felt a warmth inside and an intense gratitude for all Delia had done to help me. I wondered about her sense of duty and her drive to care for others. It was more than a job. I put on my sunglasses to shield my eyes from the penetrating sun, and breathed deep, relieved to feel my strength returning.

Boniface, the driver, a native of Lusaka and new employee of the Peace Corps, turned to me and smiled. Like many Zambians, his genuine smile illuminated the space around him.

"How long will it take to get to Mulundu?" I asked.

"Fourteen, maybe fifteen hours, Miss Cherie. Depends on how many times we stop." He dodged some goats and turned the volume up on the stereo. "This is my favorite," he said. I noticed a cassette case next to me, *The Very Best of Kenny Rogers and Dolly Parton*.

Boniface sang *Islands in the Stream* clear and loud as if crooning in the shower. It was infectious. Soon, I joined in.

The song finished, and I giggled. Boniface smiled again, even wider, exposing the corner of a back tooth capped with gold.

I leaned back in my seat and watched the streets of Lusaka where men traded goods: blankets, athletic shoes, barrels of dried fish, wicker chairs, wooden carvings, plastic buckets, women's skirts, and mangoes. I felt sad as I watched from behind the glass. Poverty surrounded the city. And it only worsened the farther we drove out into the bush.

The tires kicked up the burnt red dirt from the road as we left the city and started the long journey north. Our goal: to make it to Mansa before nightfall, the capital of Luapula and the biggest town near my village, where our Peace Corps leader lived.

We stopped for a familiar lunch of millet and pumpkin leaf. While Boniface refueled the Land Cruiser, two young children approached me.

"*Umusungu, umusungu,*" they chanted.

"Hello," I said, thinking, *yes, I am white.*

The children came close and reached out their hands. They each held a small cardboard box full of candy. Shoving them closer to me, they asked, "Buy candy?"

"Candy, huh?" The closest I had come to candy during my time in Zambia was the taste of menthol. The Peace Corps provided each volunteer with a first-aid box that included a large supply of cough drops. I sucked on them like sugarcoated treats. "I'll take two."

I gave the children money and walked away, happy with my purchase. A mere twenty Kwacha, equivalent to less than a penny, for Snickers bars. I climbed back into the Land Cruiser and we headed off down the road. I looked at Boniface and smiled.

"What is it?" he asked.

"I bought chocolate for us."

"Chocolate?"

"Yes, one for you," I said, feeling proud, handing him the candy bar, "and one for me."

"Thank you, Miss Cherie."

My senses heightened, ready to celebrate the sweetness of sugar, and the smooth, rich flavor of chocolate. I opened the wrapper and stared at the prize in my hand. It was moving. Moving?

Hmm. That's odd. It must be melting. Better eat it quickly.

I brought the candy up to my mouth. The outside layer of the milk chocolate bulged. It had a hole in the center; a large hole. I broke the bar in half to find four maggots crawling in between the layers of nougat, caramel, and peanuts.

I turned to Boniface who opened his mouth to take a bite. "No!" I grabbed the candy bar from him.

"What's wrong?"

"Maggots!" I showed him my candy bar. "Pull over!" I shouted.

Those cream-colored maggots looked suspiciously similar to the ones that came out of my butt months ago. I wondered if they sought revenge for what I had done to their buddies down in southern Zambia. Maybe they had some sort of maggot organization and I was on their wanted list.

Boniface slowed and stopped on the side of the road. I wanted these things as far away from me as possible. I grabbed the candy bars and threw them into the bush, then climbed back into the Land Cruiser. Boniface shrugged and took off without saying anything, as if that kind of stuff happened all the time.

Later that afternoon, heat penetrated the windows, draining my energy. My stomach felt hollow and cramped. I adjusted my seat back, closed my eyes, and dozed off, waking a couple of hours later. Boniface drove with his eyes fixed forward navigating enormous potholes the size of boulders. I looked out my window and didn't recognize the area. Several skinny, shoeless children sucked on raw sugar cane. The women who walked beside them were shirtless, their breasts deflated, sagging to their waists. The sweat on their bodies shimmered in the harsh light of the sun.

Up ahead, two figures walked out of the tall brush alongside the road. They looked like stick figures. Two boys, barely teenagers, dressed in torn khaki uniforms with dusty black boots, glared at us. Machine guns dangled from their shoulders.

"Where are we, Boniface?"

"Zaire."

"You took the Mpeleko road? The Peace Corps told us to stay out of Zaire."

"Yes, but this will save time."

The boys with guns approached our slowing vehicle. Boniface stopped as we neared them. One boy walked up to Boniface, and the other came around to my side. Boniface rolled down his window. I kept mine up, tight, pretending it was bullet proof.

Their guns appeared dull and scuffed; that didn't minimize their menace.

Boniface spoke to the boy in Swahili. I held my breath.

The boy on my side rested his gun against the glass and stared right into me. His youthful skin was scarred, his mouth sculpted downward, his brows furrowed, and his eyes surrounded by wrinkles surprisingly deep for a boy of his age.

"Miss Cherie." Boniface tapped me on my shoulder, startling me and breaking my spell.

"What?" I pressed my hands against my chest.

"They want Kwacha."

"For what?"

"To pass."

"How much?"

"1,500 Kwacha each."

Although equivalent to two U.S. dollars, to these boys, it was a significant amount.

I leaned down, keeping my eyes focused on the boy watching me; I reached into my sock where I hid my cash. I fumbled with it, trying not to expose the wad of bills, my stipend for the entire month. I handed the money to Boniface, who handed it to the boy. He smiled and signaled to his friend, then both boys stepped back and waved us through. Boniface rolled up his window and stomped down on the accelerator.

"Don't worry," Boniface said, "they wouldn't harm us. This is the way they make money to eat."

"By threatening to kill us?"

"I am sure neither one of them has ever used those guns. It is all for show."

Tempted to look behind, I remained still and kept my gaze forward. "Do they stop everyone?"

"No."

"Then why us?"

Before Boniface could reply I answered my own question. "Because of the Peace Corps Land Cruiser, right?"

"Yes."

"And because I'm an *umusungu*, and all white people have money."

I had explained my situation to many locals before, feeling bad about the privileges I had that they did not. But by American standards, I was broke. "I'm a volunteer, not a paid employee. I have only the money the Peace Corps gives me to live on. I have nothing back home in the States."

"Even so, to them you are rich."

I knew he was right. I took a deep breath. The cadence of my heart had almost returned to a regular, steady beat. As scared as I had been, I now felt more guilt than fear.

In Mansa, Boniface dropped me off at the Peace Corps leader's house, where I stayed for a few days to recuperate further before returning to my village.

While there, three other volunteers visited from their villages to get supplies. We shared stories about our physical and mental acclimations. Our leader assured us that every volunteer experienced these types of changes, and our bodies would adjust.

I chose to believe him.

The day before traveling back to Mulundu, I was gazing at the okra in a fly-infested produce stand in the town marketplace when I met a man, a local of Mansa. His arms hung lanky, his face long, his bald head smooth.

He glanced at me with a smile. Guarded, I half smiled back. Rape was common in Zambia, more common than a child living past the age of five. I needed extra vigilance. I didn't know who he was or what he wanted.

"Hello, miss. My name is Teddy," he said.

"*Mulishani mukwai*," I said.

He laughed. "Oh, you speak some Bemba," Teddy said in surprisingly good English. "I am well, thank you. Are you one of the Peace Corps?"

"Yes. I'm Cherie. I am stationed in Mulundu."

"Miss Cherie, I am thankful to meet you. Your Peace Corps group is welcome here. I work for the LADDC, the Luapula Association for Disabled and Disadvantaged Children. It is a shame. Difficult to receive funding to help the children." Two flies walked across Teddy's face up to his head. Never once did he shoo or swat at them.

I had heard of this organization before. I started to feel more at ease. "I know it must mean a lot to their parents, knowing someone cares." I handed him 1,500 Kwacha.

"Oh, thank you, thank you. It is difficult to make people understand why they should help."

"I know, Teddy. Everyone's so busy taking care of their own needs, their own problems. I can't blame them for that. I'm running into this situation in my village trying to gain support for my projects. Do you ever get frustrated?"

"No." Kindness illuminated his eyes, a powerful reflection of hope.

"I wish I could say the same." I sighed. "I just started my work, and already it feels like there are so many obstacles, like funding and not many people willing to help. I sometimes doubt my ability to make a difference."

Teddy selected the least damaged mango, brought it up to his nose and inhaled, then set it down and replaced it with a second mango. "You will accomplish what you need to, when you need to. As long as you believe you can, you will make a difference. That is how I feel, and that keeps me going." He placed his hand on his heart and patted his chest.

"Are you always this positive?"

"I try. I see it in this way. Who knows where I'll be in a year from now? I might be handicapped and needing someone to lend a hand. These kids need someone. I will be that someone." Teddy grinned. I could sense his genuine conviction. It energized me.

I never saw him again, but my sense of belonging to a greater good saturated my thoughts. It felt good to see locals also trying to improve their conditions. Like we were all in it together.

The next day on the ride to my village, I realized I was on a roller coaster of optimism and pessimism. Teddy had helped me reach a summit. I thought about why I felt destined to help people whose needs were greater than mine. I believed in the words of a Welsh activist named Wilfred Grenfell: "The service we render others is the rent we pay for our room on earth."

chapter five

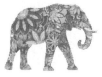

DIGGING
MYSELF A HOLE

MAY 1994 – ZAMBIA

Almost a week had passed. I finished my antibiotics and settled into village life back in Mulundu. I had missed the quiet, desolate scenery, the rows of mud huts, and the Chipilis, especially Fewdays. He greeted me with his hands clasped together and a warm expression. I felt pleased to return and ready to help.

I was not a religious person. Often I doubted the existence of a higher power, but attending church was an earnest way to master more of the language, meet more of the community, and encourage the villagers to get involved with my work.

On the Sunday after my return, I attended church service for the first time with the Chipilis. The Christian church, a small mud-brick building with a thin layer of thatch for a roof, had holes in the bricks for ventilation. The door at the back consisted of a large, rough opening. The inside was bare except for chairs and a lopsided lectern. The hot air felt oppressive and smelled like sweat.

The congregation of about forty people, the majority of whom had only heard of my presence in their village, welcomed me by asking me to stand, and then clapped in unison three times, a sign of esteem. A representative spoke to me in Bemba slowly enough for me to understand, welcoming me and wishing me a pleasant and healthy stay in Zambia. I sat, feeling embarrassed and overwhelmed. A surge of warmth filled my chest and I held back tears.

For the first time since arriving, I believed I belonged in Mulundu and my presence would be beneficial to the village, even though many people continued to stare at me throughout the service.

As I had learned is customary in any church service, religious ceremony, or funeral in Mulundu, the women wrapped their hair up on their heads as a sign of respect for God. The men sat on the left side of the church, and the women and children on the right.

During the service, I only understood some of what was being said, partially since everyone spoke in Bemba, but also because I felt hot, dizzy, and faint. My stomach cramped, and I tensed, trying to keep my composure. It helped when it came time to sing, since I distracted myself by following along with the written-out hymns.

I had attacks of intense stabbing stomachaches and light-headedness that increased over the next few weeks, but I felt determined to work. With the help of Fewdays and some of the local council members, I began work on two latrines on the outskirts of the village, one latrine for the men, another for the women. My plan called for a three-meter-deep hole, one meter in diameter, covered by a concrete slab with a nine-inch hole in the center, surrounded by a basic structure of mud brick with a large plastic pipe on top for ventilation.

I postponed work on my own personal latrine to finish these first. The community deserved this, and I wanted everyone to see my progress and perhaps pique their curiosity so they might participate in future projects.

On one scorching day, while Fewdays and I dug a hole for a latrine, I'd realized that we had been working for four days straight. Only Fewdays and I actually ever dug. It made me wonder: Why am I working so hard to help these people if they aren't willing to help themselves?

A council member stopped by to check on our progress. He could not stay and chat since he was on his way to a funeral. Each time I greeted someone, they were either on their way to or coming from a funeral. When the council member left, I thrust my shovel into the ground and grunted.

"What is it, Miss Cherie?" Fewdays said.

"This needs to stop."

"You want me to stop digging?"

"All of these deaths. It has to stop. It has to stop!" I remembered why I wasn't religious. I could not comprehend how there could be such suffering if God existed. It made no sense. No sense at all.

"I know this. But you are here now. We are digging. We will make these latrines, and they will help. Then we can start on the wells."

"But everything takes so much time. We can't move fast enough. There are so many people who need help now and there are only two of us."

Fewdays placed his hand on my shoulder. "You know we are planning to talk at the next council meeting. You will speak. They will listen. We will recruit people to help. You'll see."

I looked at him. His eyes expressed hope. "You're right. Let's keep digging."

Fewdays smiled. I studied him, standing in this hole with me, digging in the blistering afternoon sun. His face was warm and radiant, like sunshine. He was a gentle soul, a person I was lucky to know. He had more faith in me than I ever had in myself. I thought about his name, and how his father said Fewdays had always been frail. Though he received a small stipend from the Peace Corps to house and support me, I could see he worked from a place of kindness. And he was anything but frail. His spirit was mighty and his sense of purpose, to care for his family, his fellow villagers, and now me, unwavering.

Perspiration collected on the sides of my face and neck as I plunged my shovel into the ground. My stomach ached, and my legs felt limp. I ignored them and worked through the discomfort thinking about all of the people I had met thus far in my village, their gracious ways, their poverty, and their disease. Humbled, my heart felt like a sponge, absorbing every life lesson I could.

A clean bottle of water, a pair of sturdy shoes, and a meal without insects crawling into the pot were now luxuries. A day without the bell tolling was an extraordinary day.

Other than building wells and latrines, and addressing basic hygiene and sanitation issues in the village, Fewdays and I agreed to exchange cultural and linguistic knowledge. I never thought to ask Fewdays where he learned to speak English, but his vocabulary overflowed with clichés, usually placed at inappropriate moments in our conversation. A striking example occurred one night after dinner when Fewdays updated me on the news from around the village.

"And some more sad news today," he said, his tone serious. "There is a woman in the next village about my age, and she has been ill. And today she finally kicked the bucket. She just croaked."

Although this was nothing to joke about, I couldn't contain my laughter. I pretended there was something in my throat, so I reached for my water bottle and took a swig. "I'm sorry, Fewdays, but those phrases you used, they're, well, it's difficult to explain." I giggled. "They aren't quite appropriate for delivering such somber news."

"Okay. Please tell me."

We talked late into the star-filled night about communication and the pitfalls of learning a new language. I explained what clichés were, and that I noticed he used them all the time, phrases like: "practice makes perfect," "what will be will be," "out of the blue," and my favorite, "after I throw in the towel of politics."

"Fewdays, how do I sound, speaking in Bemba?"

"Good," he said without hesitation.

"Really? I think I must sound silly, because each time I speak people laugh, and I'm not trying to be funny."

Fewdays chuckled. "They are happy."

"They are happy when I speak?"

"Yes, that too."

"Ah, so, they laugh because I sound ridiculous, or because I'm a foreigner trying to speak their language?"

"It is the second one." Fewdays flashed a wide and forthright grin.

I wasn't convinced. Even so, Fewdays was kind to me and never would have let me believe I sounded silly.

I figured I was doing something productive in my village—making people laugh. Although their laughter was partially at my expense, it didn't bother me. I felt pleased to make them happy in any way I could.

I had only been working five days when my symptoms flared. I started to weaken once again, and my stomach became uneasy. I hitched a ride from a family traveling to Mansa to start another course of Flagyl. I spent three days there, resting and regaining my strength.

"I'm ready to go back to my village again," I said to Roger, the Peace Corps leader, who took care of me while I convalesced in Mansa. His house stood twice as large as the Chipilis, adorned with wicker furniture and several empty bottles of Fanta and the local beer, Mosi, strewn across the kitchen counter.

"You sure, girl? You don't seem well enough to go back to your village yet," Roger said with his Virginian accent as he slicked back his straggly hair with his hand.

"I need to get back in time for the council meeting. Fewdays is counting on me." I looked at Roger's bright, tie-dyed T-shirt and felt dizzy.

"If ya say so, but I think you'd be best to stay another night."

"I'll be fine, Roger, don't worry."

I hitched a ride on a truck filled with chickens and goats, and once again returned to my village.

Two days later, I attended the much anticipated council meeting with Fewdays. It was being held to discuss the location of the new village marketplace and the work Fewdays and I were doing on the latrines. This was exciting progress and an important meeting since it showed people were getting involved. It was held in an open dirt field on a dry and sweltering afternoon. Thirty people attended. We sat in wooden chairs facing a row of similar chairs occupied by the head chief of the village and a handful of dignified elder council members. None of them smiled. Their dark faces melted together in the harsh sunlight, but I could see their eyes staring out into the crowd like animals observing their prey.

It was a tumultuous time in Mulundu. The death toll from disease was escalating. Suicides were on the rise. Many men found less shame in hanging themselves or wandering off into the bush than in facing a long, drawn-out illness in front of their families. The head chief of Mulundu was also dying. There would soon be a change in power.

The searing sun beat down on my face as I listened to the newest council member. My stomach contracted, and I doubled over. I struggled to keep upright in my chair, but each time I tried, I felt like I had been kicked in the abdomen by a rabid kangaroo.

Not again. Not here, not now. Please let me get through this meeting.

My body had its own agenda, and being at this community meeting was not on it.

I leaned over to Fewdays and whispered, "I'm sorry, but I'm having another attack. I need to leave."

"Do you need help?" he whispered back.

"No. Stay. Speak on my behalf. We can discuss this later. I'm sorry."

"Don't worry. All will be fine. Go."

I half stood, gripping my stomach, and stepped slowly past the others across the dirt field toward the village. I wanted to find somewhere private, but I wasn't familiar with this area. Children who kicked an old torn-up shoe along the road eyed me. Women balanced large buckets of water on their heads as they walked back from the river.

I didn't know where I was headed, but I needed to get there fast. The stabbing in my stomach intensified. I held my abdomen with both hands, started to spin, stumbled, and fell onto the ground. I wasn't going anywhere. My stomach shot out a series of forceful pangs, and my underwear filled up with fluid stool. And then I passed out.

It took Fewdays almost an hour to find me.

"Miss Cherie?" He put his hand on my shoulder.

I groaned, half conscious.

Fewdays recruited another man, and they carried me to the village medical clinic, a tiny structure without solid doors or windows. I had seen it before. There was no trained medical staff, only a couple of villagers who volunteered. It had tiny mattresses, three metal bins of used needles, a couple of basins with murky water, a pile of cloth bandages, a basket of pill bottles, and a random pile of other unsanitary supplies.

"No. Not there!" I screamed.

Fewdays tried to calm me. "You can go and rest. We can give you some medicine."

"No. Please take me home. We'll get a message to the Peace Corps somehow. They'll help."

"That is too far."

"Please, Fewdays, don't take me in there."

"As you wish, Miss Cherie. We'll take you to see a friend."

They carried me to an elderly woman's house in the next village. She was a Scottish missionary and nurse named Rose; her clothes belonged in the 1940s, and her strong, sweet voice to a choir. She agreed to take care of me until the Peace Corps sent someone to help.

My arms and legs felt limp and lifeless. I couldn't catch my breath. It felt like I was falling down a dark, desolate hole, alone. I could no longer pretend to possess strength. I was in agony, and I was afraid.

For two days, Rose did her best to care for me, rubbing cool towels across my face that smelled like lavender, reading me poetry from Yeats and Wilde, and stories of Mary, Queen of Scots. I faded in and out of consciousness.

I saw a figure appear in the doorway near the foot of my bed. I focused, not trusting my eyes. "Boniface, is that you?"

"Yes. I'm here to take you to Lusaka." He reached out to help me out of bed. "Miss Cherie, you do not look good."

"Nice to see you too, Boniface."

He helped me into the Land Cruiser. I put my backpack on the floor and leaned my head back as Boniface took off down the road on the start of another fourteen-hour ride.

Something foul permeated the air. My nostrils flared. What was that stench? I looked beside me, and in the center seat between us sat a large box of uncovered dried fish.

"What's with the fish?"

"Ah. I got this from a man at the open market in Mansa. A good price too." He lifted his chin and grinned.

The heat combined with the smell of the fish intensified my nausea. I dared not ask him to part with the sardine-like creatures since he boasted about bringing them back for his family. I kept quiet and endured the heinous smell, which forced us to make several stops along the roadside as I alternated between throwing up and answering the assertive calls of nature.

It was almost midnight on a Friday when we arrived at Delia's house. I slept through the night in her spare room, and on Saturday morning Kyle, the country director, picked me up and brought me to his home. A tall, handsome man with round glasses and salt-and-pepper hair, Kyle was a Peace Corps veteran and had seen his share of illness. He parked his truck in the driveway of his house, which mimicked a compound, fenced off by barbed wire, and had a booth with a night watchman.

"You can stay in my guest house. It's small, but private."

I was delirious, tired, and unmotivated to speak. Kyle helped me into the guest house, a tiny detached bungalow with a twin bed, a wooden crate with a lamp on it, a portable fan, and a small window with brown curtains. I forced myself under the blanket on the bed and closed my eyes.

"I'll take you to the doctor on Monday. Try and rest. I'll be inside if you need me."

I slept through the weekend, eating little and talking with no one.

chapter six

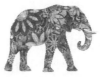

NOT SO YOUNG
OR INVINCIBLE

MAY 1994 – ZAMBIA

Sitting in the hospital in a small examination room Monday morning, I couldn't remember any dreams from my weekend of sleep or anything much at all. I surveyed the room: a table with medical supplies, a stack of unmarked boxes, and yellowed posters with torn corners depicting African children being given immunizations. Acid rose in my throat as I imagined all the used needles transmitting disease. The feeling of being watched brought me back to the moment.

"Good morning, Cherie. I'm Dr. Bush," he said with a pleasant South African accent. "Kyle told me what you've been going through. Let's see if we can figure this out, shall we?" His skin looked pale and clear like tissue paper, his expression pensive.

A rhetorical question. Good. I didn't answer. I sat hunched over on the examination table. Dr. Bush conducted a thorough examination and requested a number of tests.

A leggy, dark-skinned nurse dressed in white came in and prepared to take my blood.

"Before you do that, may I see the package, please?" I had never been afraid of needles. But in Zambia I was.

"Of course." The nurse showed me a needle encased in a sealed plastic package.

"Okay, that's fine. Thanks."

Her expression didn't change, as if mine was not the first request of this kind. When she finished, I stood to leave, and the doctor came back.

"I doubt this will show anything, but to be safe, let's do a malaria smear; that way we'll have checked most everything. Nurse, please take care of that." Dr. Bush patted me on the back, and then walked out saying, "I'll see you in a couple days."

I made it through the next forty-eight hours with Delia's help, lots of rest, and copious amounts of treated, clean water. My symptoms eased, and I had enough energy to make my own breakfast. Kyle was busy working, so Delia drove me to see Dr. Bush.

Back in his office, the air felt stale and hot. I took a couple of deep breaths and stared at the posters on the walls, this time noticing the light reflected in the eyes of the children. It looked like hope.

Dr. Bush entered the room and sat across from me. "I have your results."

"And?"

He wiped a bead of sweat from his furrowed brow. "All of the tests came back negative."

After a long pause, Dr. Bush continued. "Except that malaria slide. That came back positive."

My chest tightened. "Malaria?"

"I'm afraid so."

"H-how can that be? My symptoms don't even match those of malaria. No fever, chills, headache."

He sat next to me. "True, but in rare cases like yours that are difficult to diagnose, malaria attacks other parts of the body, like the stomach and intestines. It often goes untreated and causes a host of other problems. Cerebral malaria is another type. Be thankful you don't have that, because you'd already be dead."

I took a moment to absorb what Dr. Bush had told me. Everything looked blurry and my head started to spin, as if the diagnosis itself made me even more ill.

"But I've been so careful."

"Those anti-malarial medications you take are useful, but not one-hundred percent effective. Even if you take them as prescribed, use your mosquito netting, repellents, and so forth...." He paused, giving me a sympathetic look; "It just takes one infected mosquito, and that's it."

I looked down at my chest. My theory of doing everything I was told to prevent disease was faulty. I couldn't keep from getting sick, no matter how conscientious I was.

Dr. Bush continued, "Many of these parasites have evolved and become resistant to the preventive drugs we take. Sometimes there's nothing we can do to stop them. Not being from here, your immune system is, well, unaccustomed to dealing with these types of things."

I stayed silent.

"Stop taking the Flagyl, and we'll start you on tetracycline and quinine. Follow up with me in a few weeks."

Delia and I walked through the hospital to the pharmacy and waited for my prescriptions. She wrapped her arm around my back. We exchanged no words.

An hour later I tossed and turned in bed in Kyle's guest house with my newest prescriptions and the malaria, an accomplished assassin who had singlehandedly claimed hundreds of millions of souls.

It had gone untreated for months, and it could have been with me since I arrived five months earlier. I wanted to ask Delia if she thought I might have any long-term damage, but I already knew the answer. My body had been invaded by this pathogen for such a long time that my liver and other organs were already affected and the parasite had already replicated into thousands of new ones that had passed into my bloodstream. I understood then that I would forever carry with me my own personalized African souvenir.

I worked hard to comfort myself, comparing this latest news to the maggots-in-my-butt incident. At least now I knew.

All I wanted was sleep. I took my medications and crawled into bed thinking about the one unknown-but-mighty mosquito that had contaminated me. How many other people had she sucked blood from, stealing their vitality and leaving behind this deadly disease?

My eyelids closed, and I slept hard.

Startled awake by the intensity of a nightmare I could not recall, I opened my eyes. I saw only dark shadows in front of and all around me.

It must still be night.

I stretched my arm over to the wooden crate next to my bed and reached for my watch. My fingers explored, trying to locate it.

A repugnant, loud buzzing blared in my ears. With each second it amplified until I felt like I was being spun in rapid circles. The room and everything in it looked black. I tried to get out of bed, but fell backward and slid onto the cracked concrete floor. I pushed myself onto my hands and knees and crawled, but I could not see. Oh God. I can't see. I screamed, "Help! Kyle! Help!"

I reached one hand in front of me fumbling to find the bed, still shouting, "Help!" I don't know how loud my voice was; I couldn't hear the sounds, only muffled noises. "Why can't I hear? Why can't I see?"

Then, nothing.

Kyle rushed in and lifted me up onto the bed with a swift motion.

I turned my head and felt his warm breath on my face. I saw the faintest outline of his head. His mouth moved, but I heard nothing.

I pounded my hands on the bed and kicked my feet. "Help me!"

Kyle scooped me into his arms. I didn't know where he was taking me, but I hoped it was for medical help.

People must have been talking, birds singing, cars motoring, but for me there was only silence. There must have been shapes and colors vibrant in all directions, but for me there was only darkness.

Kyle placed me on a bed, his hand on my shoulder. I smelled disinfectant. I rocked back and forth, thinking of the malaria. Was it dying and trying to take me with it?

A cold, delicate hand touched my other shoulder, different than Kyle's. "Who's there? What do you want?"

The tender hand left my shoulder and moved up to my head and opened my right eyelid wide. A beaming flash of white appeared, then again on my left.

Minutes passed, shadows moved across the room. "What's wrong? What are you doing?"

An hour later, Kyle carried me back to his car, and darkness took me again.

"Delia, open up, it's Kyle." I could barely make out the words. They sounded drawn-out and warped. He knocked on the door with one hand, my body wilted and propped up against Kyle.

Delia opened the door, Kyle helped me inside, Delia assisted. They brought me onto her guest bed.

"Kyle, what's going on?" I vaguely heard Delia ask.

Like poor radio reception, I caught random phrases: "medications caused temporary deafness and blindness," "new prescription," "symptoms should pass."

Hours lingered. The constellation of symptoms assaulting me dissipated, and I dozed into a light slumber.

I awoke in Delia's guest bed. I yelled, "Hello?"

Delia appeared in the doorway. "You're awake. Can you hear me?" She stood in front of me.

"Yes," I said, excited.

"You've had quite the day." Delia placed a cool cloth on my forehead. A strong smell of detergent filled the air. It was a warm, muggy night, and I had been in and out of consciousness since early that morning.

I placed my hands over my heart. "That was horrifying."

"How are you now?"

"It's all still blurry, and unclear. Nothing like before. It was like being in a cave. I could only see dark shadows and hear low, distorted sounds. Like underwater."

"I can't even imagine." She paused, expressing concern. "Can I get you anything? You must be hungry." She motioned to the kitchen. "There are some leftovers from dinner."

"That would be great."

"Kyle came back to check on you and brought your things. He thought it best you stay here until you've recovered." She placed my backpack next to the bed.

"I'm sorry to impose...."

She crinkled her nose, and then smiled. "Don't mention it. I'll go heat up that food."

Delia went back to the kitchen. I grabbed my backpack and found my pen and journal.

Journal Entry

Today I will never forget, even the parts I do not remember.
I've found a new appreciation for my senses. Helen Keller
is my hero.

I scribbled with my left hand. My arm tired. I placed the journal off to the side and rested my arms on the bed. A sharp sensation shocked my right foot. I looked down and saw my toes curling under. My hands started to tremble. I couldn't stop them from moving. I sat on them, bit them, clenched them together.

Nothing worked.

My right arm shot straight out in front of me on its own like a rocket heading into space. Both of my hands thrust back and forth. My fingers coiled inward to my palms.

Oh God, what now?

"Delia!"

She sprinted into the room and stopped beside the bed. We both watched with amazement as my arms and legs collided like disharmonized percussion instruments.

Delia started to speak, and then hesitated.

"What is it?"

"It's going to be okay, Cherie, I'm calling the doctor." She ran out of the room. "Hold on."

The movements grew more powerful. I tried to swallow, but my throat constricted. I was so focused on my newest symptoms, I didn't notice Delia back at my side.

"I couldn't reach the doctor. Kyle's on his way over. Everything's going to be fine."

My legs and arms continued to shoot out against my will. Soon, my whole body was moving.

Kyle hurried into the room, eyes wide with surprise. Delia took him aside and said something in his ear, then they came to my bed. Delia tilted my head with her hand so I could see her. "I think you're having an allergic reaction to the newest medication. I need to drive to the Peace Corps office to get some medical supplies. This won't go away on its own. Kyle will stay here with you until I get back."

Kyle sat on the edge of the bed close to me. I could no longer speak and lacked any control. He held me down with one hand on my forehead and leaned over my body with his, trying to stop my haphazard motions.

"Hang on. Delia will be back soon. We'll get you through this."

I didn't believe him, and I doubted he believed it either. His eyes opened wide; perspiration formed on his brow. Tears flowed down my face.

It took Delia almost an hour to return. During that time, my body convulsed, my breathing shallowed, and I couldn't retain focus on anything except for the top half of Kyle's face. My head became cumbersome, a formidable weight I could not lift.

Kyle's head looked distorted, long and ominous. Red. Was he Satan in disguise, waiting for me to take my last breath and whisk me off to hell?

No. This was hell.

He consoled me while I searched for a way out of this agony.

I watched his eyes move up and down, felt his callused hand in my mouth, holding down my tongue, preventing me from choking.

My body jerked back and forth. I tried to keep still, but I felt exhausted. I didn't have any more strength. I no longer wanted to live. I wanted it all to end.

I reached down into my soul and prayed for death.

Please, end my suffering.

The words were bold and definite in my mind. *Please, end this.* I surrendered.

chapter seven

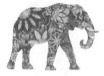

ALMOST

JUNE 1994 – ZAMBIA

Death did not come.

Delia ran into the room. Kyle kept his hand in my mouth. My arms and legs flailed. She leaned over me and looked into my eyes. Her terrified look convinced me that my wish was coming true. Both frightened and relieved, I needed this suffering to end.

They turned me onto my side, pushed the left top portion of my jeans down and stabbed me with a sharp needle.

One, two minutes, nothing.

Three, four minutes, nothing.

Five minutes, my head numbed, my feet and hands unclenched and slipped into easier positions. My neck and head sank into the pillow, and my throat relaxed, allowing me to breathe with ease.

Motionless, I gazed at Kyle and Delia and then nodded off to sleep for hours. Throughout the rest of the night, I woke terrified, my thoughts frantic, checking to see if what had happened was real, if I was alive.

I faded in and out of consciousness for days. Delia consulted with the Peace Corps physician, Dr. Enthusiasm. They stopped all of my medications. I rested. Each day I ate more and more. My nerves calmed. I felt a little stronger, but was still very tired and shocked from all that had transpired.

The Peace Corps decided I was ready for release from nursing care and sent me to a hotel for a couple of days to relax and recuperate, telling me it was important I start taking care of myself again so I could go back to my village.

"Before you go, I want to give you another malaria test," Delia said, reaching into her nursing bag for a fresh needle.

I stuck out my right hand, and she punctured my finger and retrieved a small sample of blood, which she placed on a clear, rectangular piece of plastic.

"I'll let you know what we find."

"Thanks for everything, Delia. You've been wonderful to me."

"Just doing my job."

"You saved my life. I'll never be able to thank you and Kyle enough." I held my hand over my mouth, trying not to cry.

"You can thank me by taking care of yourself. I know you don't want to hear this, but I think you should go back to the U.S. You need to recuperate."

I reached out and took her hand and squeezed it. "I understand your concern, I do. I thought I was going to die."

"You almost did."

"Okay, I almost did, but I didn't, and I'm getting stronger. I need to go back to my village." I didn't want to disappoint her, but I felt obligated to finish what I started. I couldn't quit. It wasn't in my constitution, even if malaria was now inside me.

"I don't understand why you're so compelled to go back there after everything you've been through."

I thought about why I needed to stay in Africa, despite all my problems. I remembered the haunting sound of the village church bell. I cringed.

"If I don't go back, I'll feel like I failed the people of Mulundu, and I promised Fewdays I would help. Besides, my life is not more important than a whole village. That doesn't mean I'm not afraid. I just have so much compassion for them."

"Very noble of you, but you need some help right now too. Look, I can't stop you, Cherie, but you know what I think."

"I do." I hugged her tight and said farewell.

Boniface drove me to the hotel. I spent two days wandering around the outskirts of Lusaka. I wrote in my journal, trying to capture the essence of the last few weeks, and wondered why my wish for death had not come true. Whatever the reason, I was thankful it wasn't granted.

The last malaria test came back negative. I didn't know what that meant. Was it gone? I had not finished the medications because of the complications. What about the damage left behind? And if the anti-malaria medication didn't work before, would I contract it again? What could I do to stop it? I had so many unanswered questions.

Delia told me the drugs I had taken may have eliminated the malaria, at least clinically, but I continued suffering from cramps, diarrhea, headaches, dizziness, and a host of other symptoms.

A couple of days later, I had only improved a little. I was told to get a complete physical from the Peace Corps doctor. Following the exam, the Peace Corps would decide where I was to go and what I was to do next.

"So, what exactly is going on?" inquired Dr. Enthusiasm.

"It feels like I'm shitting pine cones."

"Any other symptoms?"

"It feels like a colony of gremlins is strangling my intestines, and I have about five seconds to make it to a latrine before Mount Saint Helens erupts. I've already lost several pairs of underwear, a pair of pants, a skirt, and the remainder of my dignity."

"So…you have diarrhea?"

"Not just any diarrhea, explosive, painful, uncontrollable, and frequent diarrhea."

"Anything else?"

"Yeah, I'm dizzy, light-headed, and always tired, but I'm most concerned about the sizable amount of blood when I go."

"What color is it?"

"Ah, red, that's how I know it's blood." I became agitated. His questions seemed pointless because I didn't feel like he was going to help me. I tried to stifle my frustration.

"I'd like to do some more tests, including a rectal exam. How about tomorrow?"

"Sounds fabulous. Can't wait. Seriously, do I have a choice about this because it seems like I will be uncomfortable, considering I already feel like I have habanero peppers lining my ass, and the idea of you poking and prodding around in there doesn't thrill me."

"Sorry, the Peace Corps requires a full exam which includes the areas you're describing."

The exam felt like shards of glass being shoved up inside me. The bright red blood I saw was caused by an anal fissure—a tear in the rectum. According to the doctor, the tear looked more like the Grand Canyon.

The rest of my tests came back inconclusive. Both Dr. Enthusiasm and Delia recommended I return to the United States to undergo a thorough colon evaluation, a series of blood tests, possibly anal surgery, and, of course, convalescence.

Even after everything I had endured, I still longed to finish what I had started. But the Peace Corps, which had been so eager to get me back on my own, now told me I could not return to Mulundu until I regained my strength and fully recovered.

I had no choice but to focus on restoring my health back in the U.S., and once able, I vowed to return to Mulundu even stronger than before.

Boniface and I drove back to my village one last time to pack up my possessions and say goodbye. We drove north, and I watched the landscape of browns and tans blur together, expansive, straggly tall brush, and the orange setting sun far in the distance. Kenny and Dolly's voices blared through the speakers. I didn't sing along. Neither did Boniface.

I dreaded saying farewell to Fewdays. Despite all of the obstacles in his life, I had never seen him discouraged or doleful, but on that day, he had a deep frown and forlorn look when I told him I needed to leave.

"I want you to have all my belongings. And here," I placed my hand in his and gave him a wad of Kwacha.

"Oh, Miss Cherie, I am at a loss for words." I would miss his clichés.

"I don't want to leave, Fewdays." I gripped his hands in mine, tears forming in my eyes. "Please know that."

He squeezed my hands. His mouth turned further downward. "But you must go. You must heal. I will continue our work. The council meeting proved favorable. There will be progress. I will see to it."

"I'm so glad the meeting went well. Yes, please continue. I will return. I want to come back." I let go of his hands and hugged him. Our embrace was long and tender. Neither of us wanted to let go.

"Miss Cherie, we must get on the road. I want to get to Mansa tonight," Boniface interrupted.

"I know," I said, afraid I might never get to see the Chipilis or Mulundu again.

I hugged Agnes and Cadbury and embraced Fewdays one last time. My arms hung around his slender frame, trying to communicate my respect and fondness for him. Finally, I stepped back toward the Peace Corps vehicle and said, "I will miss you all."

"You will be fine, Miss Cherie. You will get better and then return. We will be here. Until then, we will miss you as well." His words sounded joyless, and unforgettable, and his eyes, like mine, held a sea of tears.

Boniface and I drove away from Mulundu, waving to the Chipilis and to the place I had called home. Sinking into my seat, I closed my eyes and wept all the way to Mansa, where a handful of the other volunteers had gathered for motorcycle training. I spent the night in their company, relaying my story. I had grown close with all of them throughout the initial three-month training. Our experiences together were heartfelt and not well understood by others.

In the morning, they escorted me to the vehicle where Boniface waited. Before I got in, they handed me a wooden sculpture of a hut with a family sitting in a circle and a note that read:

> "Cherie, we are all thinking about you a lot. Wishing you all the best on this. If anyone is going to turn this into a positive experience, it will be you. Your strength truly amazes us. Hear every word we say on our respect for you, since it is immense. We will be writing. Keep your strength.
>
> P.S. The sculpture celebrates all of life with freedom and energy."

I hung my head and started to cry, frightened to go home, give up on my dream, and leave all my new friends. "I'm going to miss you guys."

The other volunteers took turns hugging me. After a long farewell, I resisted breaking away from their embraces, but it was time.

I boarded the Peace Corps Land Cruiser, and Boniface and I made our last trip south to Lusaka. I stayed quiet for most of the trip, hiding behind my sunglasses and hat, trying not to let him see how broken I had become.

During the long drive, I thought about Fewdays, his parting words, his caring ways. I concentrated on what my friends had written and hoped my fellow volunteers were right. They believed in me, and I needed to believe in myself.

The flights home were long and draining for my enervated physical state. I traveled for two days, from Zambia to Zimbabwe, to Kenya, to London, then to Los Angeles.

As the plane approached LAX, I laughed as I stared out the window into the blue sky. I recalled a small booklet the Peace Corps had given us during our training, a publication titled, *A Few Minor Adjustments*, a reference to help us understand some of the mental, emotional, cultural, and even physical changes we would go through while serving as a volunteer.

What a colossal understatement. There was nothing few, minor, or merely adjustable about my time in the Peace Corps. I sensed that my mind, body, and spirit would never be the same.

I still believed I had an obligation to Fewdays and the people of Mulundu. I wanted nothing more than to regain my strength and return to Zambia to help them once again, especially since I heard that they didn't have a replacement volunteer for Mulundu.

I spent the next year undergoing medical tests and treatments. Although my symptoms improved, the Peace Corps would not allow me to go back until I had been symptom-free for over a year.

That never happened.

chapter eight

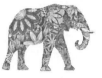

EMERGENCIES ONLY

APRIL 2004, PART II – SAN DIEGO

For over three hours, Alex and I remained hostages in our waiting-room chairs, eager to hear my name called. I leaned against him, slouched, my head on his shoulder. He stroked my hair with one hand while his other rested on my thigh. I felt relieved to have him so close, comforting me.

Alex would have been a lawyer if it weren't for his passion for computers. He was risk-averse and predominantly reclusive, the exact opposite of me. He was born and raised in New Jersey, I in Los Angeles. He excelled at calculus and financial planning; I enjoyed poetry, music, and painting abstracts.

"Thank you for being here with me," I said.

He squeezed my leg. "Don't talk, Cherie. Try and rest."

Another hour passed. "Alex, I can't wait any longer."

"I know. Hang on. I'm going to ask again." Alex hurried to the front desk.

The stench of vomit filled the air, and the sound of a thunderous cough echoed in my ears. A young blonde, plainly dressed woman two chairs away from me fought to cover her mouth as she hacked and heaved. We shared the same air. I held my breath, thinking I could become infected with a simple inhale. Bronchitis, maybe, or viral pneumonia.

Alex rushed back. "Cherie, come on." He helped me stand and escorted me into the middle of the ER.

The fluorescent lights glared into my eyes. Doctors in teal scrubs and white coats hurried back and forth. Every treatment room was full and patients lined the corridors. The nurse guided me to a gurney covered with yellowed sheets parked against a wall between two small rooms. Alex lifted me onto it, and I cradled my neck with my tired hands. Haunting moans of a woman in crisis pounded inside my mind. Surprisingly, these noises were not my own. In a room across from us an older, decrepit woman in a faded blue gown shifted haphazardly in a small hospital bed. Her pale, wrinkled skin drooped as she wailed.

Half an hour passed. Neither I nor the elderly woman had seen a doctor. Her loud laments escalated with each minute.

Her sounds both frightened and annoyed me. I wanted someone to not only ease her suffering, but to stop her insistent crying. I too felt enfeebled and overwhelmed, but I restrained my cries. I didn't know what she suffered from, and I didn't care. Unlike in Zambia when I cared much more for others than myself, I now felt consumed by my own innate desire for survival. Africa had changed me in this way too.

"Sorry to keep you waiting," a short, bald, fast-talking man said, shaking Alex's hand and nodding to me. "I'm Dr. Emergencies Only." His scarlet tie matched the color of blood.

Alex relayed what had happened to me that night and the symptoms I had been experiencing throughout the past few months: my lower-leg neuropathy, my knee instability and pain, the recent stabbing left-sided headaches, and now, my neck.

Dr. Emergencies Only fumbled through a report in his hands. "According to our records, you were seen here just two weeks ago."

I trembled as I spoke. "That's right."

He rubbed his eyes, which were bloodshot and had dark circles beneath them. He sighed then spoke, "And the doctor you saw recommended you see a cardiologist and a neurologist. Have you been to see either of them?"

Alex answered. "She hasn't yet. She saw her primary doctor, who put in requests to her insurance, but they're still pending."

After giving me a brief once-over, Dr. Emergencies Only stepped away from the gurney and folded his arms across his chest. "I realize you're in a lot of pain, and I do think there's something wrong with you. However, the ER is for trauma victims, not to diagnose long-term illnesses. I agree with the recommendations of the last ER doctor. You need to be seen by a specialist. And I don't want to prescribe pain meds since I don't know what I am treating. You can take Ibuprofen for your neck. I'm sorry. There just isn't anything else I can do for you here."

Dr. Emergencies Only hustled down the crowded hallway to attend to his next patient. I turned toward Alex. Frustration and anger surged inside me. "We waited all that time for nothing?" Again, I felt tears forming in my eyes.

He sighed and shook his head. "I'm so sorry, CK."

"Why can't he help me?"

"I think because your situation's complicated. Try not to worry. You've got that appointment with the neurologist Monday."

"That's four days away. What if he can't help me either?"

"Don't think that way. I'm sure he'll have some answers. Come on, let's get you home."

In the car, I thought about what Dr. Emergencies Only had said. To this triage specialist, my case was simple: I wasn't bleeding, having a heart attack or a stroke, and my appendages were still attached. I hadn't been shot, hit by a car, swallowed poison, or been bitten by a venomous creature. I wasn't overdosing on drugs, and my appendix and other organs were intact, but most of all, there were no tangible manifestations of my illness other than my swollen knee, crooked neck, and shortened breaths.

Before, I had believed the one place a person who felt scared and who was in extreme distress could go to for help was the emergency room. Of that, I was no longer certain.

Alex lifted me onto my bed and into my soft cotton sheets, then knelt beside me on the floor and looked in my eyes. "I'm here for you, CK. I'm going to help you get through this."

"You're such a great guy."

"Yeah, I'm not so bad," Alex said with a smirk. "Now, let's try and get some rest."

I half grinned, and half nodded. He handed me two Ibuprofen, and I swallowed hard, washing them down with a gulp of water. Alex crawled into bed next to me. I clasped his hand and watched his eyes close.

As he faded in and out of sleep, the strain in my neck and head persisted. I stared out my bedroom window into the somber sky. My midsection contracted, explosive and hard, and into the darkness of that night I wept from a place I had never experienced before. I didn't think about my job, my two cats, the sports I played, the bills on my desk, or the volunteer work I so loved, my family, or friends. Two questions plagued me: How did I get here and how would I get out?

The stillness of the night lured me deep into the melancholy of my past. I felt fortunate to have Alex by my side, unlike the other times when I suffered alone.

I remembered the second time I had wished for death and the events that brought me to that loathsome and desolate place. I thought about a man I met in New Zealand who often haunted my thoughts during those low points, like now. As independent as I was, I now thought Janis Joplin was right: freedom could indeed be just another word for nothing left to lose.

chapter nine

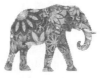

NOBODY
LOVES RAYMOND,
EXCEPT MAYBE
JACK DANIELS AND JIM BEAM

SEPTEMBER 1997 – NEW ZEALAND

Winter wasn't quite over yet, and brisk, moist winds raced across my face. I sat on a rusted metal bench at the pier in the center of Auckland waiting for the next ferry to take me to the tiny island of Waiheke, where I lived. I also waited for a dull, persistent throbbing in my head to go away. It had been over three years since my time in Africa, and I still suffered fatigue, frequent headaches, and stomach cramping.

Because the Peace Corps refused to let me return to Zambia, I had created my own adventure by moving to New Zealand. I wasn't going to let health challenges stop me. I continued to explore the world to expand my sense of freedom, and now I felt enticed by the Pacific Islands.

My body continued to communicate with me, even though I didn't know what it said. The latest was a stabbing ache in my right knee. After an X-Ray, an MRI, and several physical therapy sessions, specialists found nothing medically wrong with my knee. No doctors looked beyond the joint itself and into complications from other diseases. They agreed that malaria caused long-term damage, but nothing could be done about it, and they didn't think my knee pain was related to anything I had contracted in Africa. I assumed they knew best, so I continued with work and school.

I attributed some of my symptoms, particularly the intense fatigue, to my busy life of attending graduate school at Auckland University and working several nights a week at a wine bar to help pay my expensive overseas tuition. I rarely had time for sleep.

While sitting on the bench, the allure of the crisp, salty water rocking back and forth against the shore to one side, and the hustle of the congested city to the other, lured me into a light sleep. As I started to close my eyes, a diminutive, impressively hairy older gentleman approached me, rambling about the weather in a one-sided conversation. He sat on the ground about fifteen feet from me.

Another man, stocky and chubby around the middle, sat beside me. He looked like he had lived harder and longer than the older man. His skin was tanned a crispy brown and wrinkled, his teeth stained yellow, and his fine gray hair frayed and receding.

He leaned in to give me a closer look. "What color are my eyes, hazel or bloodshot?"

I could smell the smoke residue emanating from his clothes. "I would have to say both."

"I'm Raymond. What's your name, Pretty Eyes?"

"Cherie." There wasn't any harm in giving first names. As a traveler, some of my most surprising moments had come from staying open to the human pageant, which would never have happened if I had stayed at home and not been exposed to the unique possibilities of life.

"So, Cherie, do you get high or drink alcohol?"

"No." I returned my attention to the papers in my lap. I did not get high. I enjoyed drinking wine or beer on occasion, but it was none of his business.

"I do," he went on to say, "I've got a real problem."

I figured he was about to ask for money. I was familiar with these types of requests from strangers, especially in L.A.

"I just came from a detox center. I'm addicted to getting high and drinking." He lit up a cigarette and took a long, slow drag. "I just got out. I've been clean for a week. I'm trying. It's been an eye-opening week, Pretty Eyes."

He took another hit, and the stench of tobacco filled the air. "I've come to see a lot of things differently than I did before. I don't want to go back where I was, but I feel like I'm slipping." Raymond fidgeted, looked around. "I came down here to see if any of my mates were around. This is where we used to hang out and drink and get high. You sure I can't buy you a drink?"

"No, thank you." I wasn't sure why I kept talking to him. Maybe I sensed a common vulnerability. "I'm just waiting for the ferry."

"You a student at the university?"

"I'm completing my master's degree. In anthropology."

He pointed to some ants on the pavement below our feet. "You study insects and little creatures?"

I giggled. "Anthropology's the study of people and culture."

"Well if you're studying people, I guess my problem has to do with where I grew up. I've always been in it; I just can't get out of it. The worst part is I'm a reasonably intelligent person. I want to use my mind. I want more from this life. It makes me sad where I ended up."

I thought about how my plans to stay in Africa had been derailed and my next adventure had begun. After I returned to the U.S., I applied to graduate schools for my master's degree and was accepted to my first choice, UCLA. While waiting for my schooling to commence, I took an impromptu vacation to New Zealand. I toured the University of Auckland and, envisioning myself there, applied. Months later, I boarded a plane back to New Zealand.

Raymond continued, oblivious to my scattered thoughts. "If I keep going the way I'm going, I could end up like that guy over there." Raymond gestured to the old hairy man who sat on the ground rambling. "But I know I'm capable of more than that. What do you think?"

"I believe you are. We all are." I felt overwhelming compassion for Raymond. I had been fortunate, so many opportunities, simply by where I grew up, and the supportive family and friends I had. I wondered what I could do. Perhaps help him stay clean. Maybe even help him find some work.

His eyes opened wide. "You really think so?"

I could sense his true desire for freedom from his addiction. A hollow twinge emerged in my stomach.

"Maybe what you need is support, some people you can talk to, people who are not addicts. Do you have anyone to help you?"

"They're all into drugs and alcohol like me. That's one of my problems." He took another puff on his cigarette. "Have you heard of Alcoholics Anonymous?"

"I have. Perhaps they can help you," I said, still hopeful I would get the courage to offer my friendship.

"They did. That's how I've been clean for seven straight days."

"That's great. You should stick with it." I wanted to offer my help, but I didn't know him. I needed to be cautious.

"I think I need to hit rock bottom first. I've been close a few times, but I've never been there. I think I need to get badly hurt before I get out of this."

The ache in my stomach grew. "I hope that's not true."

Raymond glanced over at the papers on my lap.

"Can I write something for you?"

"Sure." I handed him my pen and a blank sheet of paper.

"You won't like what I write. It will make you sad." He wrote each letter as if he were creating a masterpiece. "What are you studying now?"

"A paper on seasonal affective disorder."

"Seasonal what?"

"It's a type of depression."

"I know about that. Self-pity. I'm a weak person. When I think about the weak person I am, I need something to take me away, but even while I'm high, I can't get away from it. It's scary; depression.

It sneaks up on you, and before you know it, you picture yourself jumping off the Auckland Bridge."

"You aren't going to...."

"Not today, but as I mentioned, with depression, you never know. That's why I need a drink. I have to get out of my head."

Small brown birds gathered around the sidewalk beside us, searching for food, hurrying from one morsel to the next. I thought about Raymond and his depression and pictured him jumping from a bridge with no one noticing he was gone.

Raymond finished writing and handed back my paper and pen. I searched for something comforting to say, but although I studied depression, I had never faced anything like what he described.

I contemplated steering him away from his focus on alcohol and asking him to go get a cup of tea, but strange men unnerved me. I didn't think he meant me any harm, but I didn't know for certain.

The ferry arrived, and I got up to leave.

The old hairy guy stumbled back over to me and said, "That there's the ferry to Waiheke."

"Yes, thank you."

I placed the pad of paper and pen in my backpack and swung the bag over my shoulder. Raymond stood and said, "Good luck with your studies, Pretty Eyes."

"Thanks. Good luck to you too. What are you going to do now?"

He looked at me, frowned and said, "I'm going to get a drink. I don't have any other choice. I just wish I had someone to drink with. I hate drinking alone."

I found a seat inside the ferry. Across from me was a tiny concession stand where people waited in line to purchase wine or beer.

I could sure use a drink.

I thought about Raymond. His urge to drink. I had the discipline to resist and turn on and off my indulgences, at least when it came to drinking, but I possessed another type of addiction: envy. Although I didn't envy rich, powerful, or famous people, or crave anything material, I envied those who were healthy. I longed to feel

71

as good as I had before my time in Africa. It felt exhausting, carrying around my desire to be something other than what I was. Maybe that was how Raymond felt.

The ferry disembarked, and I remembered Raymond's message. I scrambled through all of the stray papers in my bag and found his words, written in all capital letters.

"THE STOMACH OF SOCIETY HAS FOUND ME INDIGESTIBLE. AND SO NOW I REMAIN A PRISONER IN THIS RECEPTACLE OF VOMIT."

Raymond was right. His words did make me sad. I had never felt that type of loneliness or internal despair before, but one day I would.

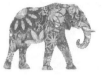

chapter ten

PHARMAWHATICALS

SPRING 1998 – SAN DIEGO

Twenty-seven years old, I had completed my master's degree months earlier. After graduating, I had moved from New Zealand to San Diego, the city where I had completed my bachelor's degree before going to Zambia. During my time in Auckland, I had missed California, the place where my family and closest friends lived. New Zealand kept me warm with fond memories, but San Diego was where I felt I belonged.

Relocating to Southern California proved challenging. I had no money, no job, and no idea what to do next.

To help with my search for employment, I bought my first car, a well-used—over 160,000 miles—Mitsubishi Colt for the negotiated price of $750. Although I got my U.S. driver's license at age sixteen, my international driver's license at age twenty, and my New Zealand driver's license by twenty-four, I had never owned a car. I biked everywhere I could, and if I couldn't walk or bike, I took a bus, borrowed a friend's car, or boarded a train.

I had oddly delighted in being without a vehicle and loathed the day I would purchase one. I did not want to end up like every other Southern Californian who relied on their car. Now that I owned one, it would not own me. I would still cycle and walk to as many places as I could. Back in California, I relearned how to drive on the right side of the road and soon realized that sixty-five was the new fifty-five on most major freeways.

Other minor adaptations included not being able to purchase a large bag of kiwi fruit for a dollar, or find my favorite New Zealand wines and other delicacies like pumpkin soup and kumara chips. I also missed taking in the breathtaking hills of green alongside the deserted beaches that stretched along New Zealand's spectacular landscape after an afternoon of sailing or playing touch rugby with friends. But my newest challenge soon became evident. For the first time, I had no idea what my next steps were. My Type A personality floundered. I was, by choice, a product of academia and adventure, and even though I had worked since I was sixteen to supplement my education, I no longer had any specific goals for higher learning, travel, or vocation, which I had always relied on to protect myself from myself.

With no income and deep in debt from my expensive overseas graduate school, I found employment as a bartender in Cardiff at a restaurant a few paces from the sand that nuzzled up against the Pacific Ocean. I often worked seven days a week, ten-hour days, paying off my debt while deciding what to do next. There wasn't much demand for anthropologists in San Diego. When I embarked on my studies, I realized the need for experts in this field of work was slim, even within an academic setting, but as a citizen of the world, I wanted to understand the global culture I lived in. I didn't want practicality to stop me from doing something I loved. Though my formal studies were complete, I continued to crave knowledge, to understand deeper our existence as human beings, so I applied for a Ph.D. program, which would be my next great enterprise.

I organized a meeting with the head of the department at the University of California at San Diego and brought my transcript and diploma, recommendations from three of my undergraduate professors, a certificate stating the training and work I had completed while in the Peace Corps, and a letter from the Country Director explaining why I didn't complete my service. I also had a copy of my diploma from my master's program, a copy of my dissertation, and three recommendations from professors I had studied under at the University of Auckland.

"Cherie, a pleasure to meet you," said Dr. Culture, the head of the Anthropology Department. Her face looked stern but youthful, clothes meticulous, and her auburn hair tied in a ponytail. Artifacts from Africa and South America adorned her office. A collection of wooden masks filled one wall and a large framed map of the world hung behind her polished teak desk.

I reached out and shook her hand. "Thank you for meeting with me. I'm excited about continuing my education here at UCSD."

She pointed to a chair. "Have a seat."

I sat and handed her my documents, explaining their relevance one by one.

She flipped through them, smiling, nodding, genuinely pleased with everything.

"It looks to me like you're more than qualified to return to us for graduate work in anthropology. However, we have strict rules in this department."

"What do you require? A thesis proposal? Entrance exam?"

"You must possess a master's degree in anthropology from this university. I would be happy to admit you to the master's program. Upon completion you could continue on to your Ph.D."

"But I already have a master's degree."

"Yes, your credentials are quite impressive, receiving first class honors. You're definitely qualified."

"And I can bring real-world experience, having lived overseas, traveled to many different countries, and studied different languages...."

"Considering everything, instead of a two-year commitment to the master's program, we could waive the first semester of the first year. That way you would only have to take the second semester classes, and complete the second year with a thesis."

A knot formed in my stomach. "With all due respect, I've already written a dissertation and completed four full semesters of graduate classes."

She interlaced her fingers and rested her arms on the desk. "I know, I'm sorry, Cherie, but we require everyone to go through these necessary prerequisites. This is not in any way personal against you, or the education and experience you have."

I glanced at the masks. One of them had a sinister grin. "There isn't anything else you can do?"

"I'm afraid not, but I do hope you will consider the option we discussed since you would be a nice addition to our program." She handed back all of my papers, on top of which sat her business card. She shook my hand, wished me luck, and escorted me to the elevator.

I thanked her for her time, entered the elevator, and as the doors shut, I screamed. On the way to my car, I felt her business card in my hand and threw it in a dumpster.

I thought about returning to New Zealand for my Ph.D., but that was only a fleeting idea. I wanted to remain in San Diego. I didn't know what else to do. Besides bartending nights and weekends, I began working full-time as a writer and editor for a non-profit organization to make ends meet.

Suddenly, my brain chemistry shifted. I became pensive, believing my life had no meaning. Without a clear direction and something to accomplish, I could no longer prove to myself, and the world, that I was worthy of love and worthy of life. My perfectionism stabbed at me like demented daggers.

Never before had I understood rage. Now, I encountered it, deep in every part of me. I hated myself and who I had become. Without anything to achieve, I was not good enough for anyone, but most of all, I was not good enough for my biggest critic: myself.

I was young, educated, well-traveled, and relatively healthy—some of my symptoms from my time in Africa had been remedied by persistence with a healthy diet, rest, exercise, and of course, through the benefits of youth. I embraced and loved life. But none of that mattered. At night I locked myself in my bedroom, away from my roommate, away from the world, cradling my pillow, swaying backward, then forward on my bed, as if in a trance.

My journal became my closest companion and what felt like my only one. It did not offer advice, scold, or lecture me. It listened to my desperation.

The darkness inside me begged for release. My hand cramped trying to keep up with my thoughts, scribbling nearly illegible words across pages and pages, every night for weeks, sometimes until dawn.

Journal Entry

All the doors of life appear closed. I feel trapped in a life, a mind, a vision of confusion and isolation. My heart is drenched with black. What more can I give to continue beating these persistent demons? They fight and wear me down. I am wretched, nothing. I am no one. The demons, they are victorious. Please deliver me from this horrid pain. Carry me away. No. Let me deliver myself.

I had no answers for my lost soul. My journal turned on me. Its once kind and hospitable pages were now evil, luring me in to my self-destructive thoughts and malicious mind.

Biking home from work in Cardiff at midnight, I trembled with panic, believing that soon I might cause serious harm to myself. I needed to stay away from my house, my room, my journal—that ominous object, its energy and influence, fiercer than my own, no longer my ally.

Light rain filled the air. My hands shook as I stopped at a store and picked up a shopping basket. Walking up and down the aisles, my eyes glossed over the shelves.

I can't live like this anymore.

I dropped the plastic basket on the tile floor and ran out crying. I hopped on my bike and rode up Coast Highway, pushing hard on the pedals, running red lights, screaming and wailing out into the cloudy night sky with my helmet tied to my backpack and the switch on my bike light off.

I flung my arms up into the air and shouted, "I'm so sorry. I can't do this any longer." I rode across three lanes of sparse traffic to the other side of the street, half hoping a car would take me away with one fell swoop. No more anguish, just blackness.

A horn blared and a white pickup swerved around me. I felt the rush of wind as it passed. I didn't care. I continued to steer my bike back and forth through the lanes, the brine of tears mixed with the rain clouding my vision. Another car barreled by. My heart hammered. My legs moved in swift circles, propelling me across the street onto Moonlight Beach. I tossed my bike onto the sand and dashed into the white water up to my waist. Minutes later, I stood, soaking and shivering, watching my tears disappear into the murky water. I tilted my head back and reached my arms out toward the luminous moon, begging for freedom from my agony.

Dive in, Cherie. You'll float out to sea. It will be gentle.

My arms shivered but my legs froze in the movement of the waves and the penetrating cold of the water, reflected by the brightness of the moon.

I did not understand my suffering, but as I examined the beaming light of the moon, I thought about the vast universe, picturing the multitude of stars, planets, and beings thriving, not by themselves, but intermingled with each other.

I observed the water, stretching out for so many miles, all the way to the Pacific Islands, and remembered Raymond. It wasn't society that found me repulsive and indigestible—I managed to do that all by myself.

Somewhere at my core, standing in that frigid water, breathing deep beneath the moon, I realized I had worked so hard to create a life of value and joy, one that I could be proud of. I thought about several friends who had died before the age of twenty-six. Cynthia from skin cancer. Jin killed by a train. Renee drowned. Kristi hit by a car while crossing a street. Taylor jumped off an overpass onto a busy highway. And Mick, my closest friend whom I had met while studying in England, was a peaceful, all-creature-loving vegetarian.

He adored everyone and everyone adored him. He was murdered by a stranger who robbed, beat, and set him on fire in a deserted rural barn.

I cried for my fallen friends and the injustice of the human condition and wept for how I felt shackled by self-loathing. I had to find a way to alleviate my mental anguish and live, if not for me, for all of my friends who were no longer able to experience the wonders of this world.

Backing out of the water, I collapsed onto the wet sand, and cried in a fetal position until I ran out of tears. I straightened my legs. Wiped the wet sand from my face. Announced to the night, "Enough."

Because of my HMO insurance, it took weeks to get a consultation with Dr. Dedicated-to-Drugs, a gray-haired psychiatrist who was kind, quirky, and acted as though he knew me well. He was the type of guy that everyone liked, a great conversationalist, with the smooth voice of a deejay, and a politeness that rivaled Mr. Rogers.

Please, won't you be my patient?

The décor of his office matched his disposition; bright yellow, landscape pictures of meadows and diplomas on the walls, and two plastic plants flanked a tall, slender bookshelf filled with reference books.

We talked for hours, session after session, about my feelings, my childhood, my experiences, and the layers started to fall away. After six sessions, he gave me a series of tests to understand my depression and innermost feelings. I had no prior experience with therapy and doubted someone I had just met could understand me when I didn't even know myself.

Following a combination of oral and written examinations, I took my fourth and final test on a computer that was a time-sensitive exam that monitored and recorded both my answers and reactions. I felt anxious, as if in school, wanting to excel at everything. I wanted to perform well (whatever that meant, since there were no right or wrong answers), and to show my aptitude.

The overzealous part of me that needed to show the world I was tough and capable should have been the psychiatrist's biggest clue, but I wasn't ready to divulge that information. I believed it was my personality, wanting to do my best at everything. What was so wrong with that?

"Cherie, come on back," Dr. Dedicated-to-Drugs said with a polite smile and huge wave. He always wore khaki pants, a collared shirt, and the same tweed blazer.

I leaped out of the waiting-room chair and followed him to his office. He closed the door and waved for me to take a seat. Waving was a big thing for him.

It had been two weeks since I had taken those tests. I felt jittery and ready to hear my results.

"I'm sure you're wondering about your tests," he said.

"Yes. And?" I felt like I was in kindergarten again, ants in my pants, waiting for the teacher to give me my first report card.

"All of your tests, coupled with the information from our first few discussions, lead me to believe you have something called Attention Deficit Hyperactivity Disorder, better known as ADHD."

"Isn't that a disorder only found in children?"

"There are several adults who were never diagnosed as children and have attempted to cope with this disorder without knowing it. Most people with ADHD have trouble paying attention and are easily distracted. They have a difficult time focusing and are unorganized. Because of their low attention span, they often cannot complete tasks."

"I've finished everything I've attempted and I'm quite organized."

"I'm certain that's true, which brings me to the next set of symptoms: hyperactivity and impulsivity. Some adults, with lots of discipline and practice, battle their distractibility and manage their lives by focusing on their strengths, since many people with ADHD are intelligent and creative. They do what I call hyper-focusing."

Curious, I waited for him to explain.

"People are able to channel their hyperactive energy into something they are passionate about, often going overboard on new challenges, and throwing themselves into situations without critical thought, logic, or judgment. Unfortunately, once their interest fades on that subject, they move on to the next most interesting thing, whether it's a new job, relationship, or place to live. People with this mass of energy frequently feel restless and are unable to relax."

The word relax hadn't quite finished echoing in the room when our eyes met. We both gazed down at my right knee bobbing up and down in tiny uncontrolled motions.

"Cherie," he continued, "do you remember the last test you took on the computer that asked for certain responses?"

"Yes."

"That test analyzes your reaction time to a variety of stimuli. Every one of your answers was premature, meaning you reacted before you had all of the information. The test was designed to study your level of hyperactivity and impulsiveness. You had a perfect score, leaving me little doubt about how this part of your brain functions."

Maybe I was hyperactive and spontaneous, but there was something even more telling: I moved around a lot, loved trying new things, and changing almost everything and anything, from types of spaghetti sauce to residences. Even relationships. I thrived on change, but never thought there was something wrong with me. I had always embraced it as who I was. What did that say about my accomplishments? Was I merely a by-product of a disorder? Did that diminish who I had become?

"You're a competent and ambitious young woman. That's why you have done so well for yourself, but I do believe one of the reasons you're depressed is because the coping mechanisms you have used throughout your life are no longer working. You get angered easily and sometimes act before thinking, right?"

"Recently, yes. And it's happening more and more."

"This isn't something you can control on your own. I think it best to prescribe some medication called Ritalin. It can be effective for treating the symptoms you're exhibiting."

"Hmm. Okay."

"In the meantime, let's see each other every two weeks."

I left, fidgety and anxious. I didn't want to take medication, but I didn't see another choice. I filled my prescription and drove to the nearest bookstore, where I flipped through a large variety of books: ADD/ADHD in Children, ADHD in Adults, ADHD in Women, ADHD and Relationships, ADD and Learning Disabilities, ADD and Work. I was surprised there wasn't a book for ADHD and People Who Knit.

I couldn't decide which one to purchase, so I bought them all. Thirteen books and over $300. The clerk at the counter looked at every title as he swiped the barcode. After about the eighth book, he looked at me with a smirk, as if I was the fourteenth book in the stack, ADHD and Impulsivity Exemplified.

I tried to halt his suspicions by threading my lying needle. "I'm doing a research project."

"Uh huh."

Once home, I spread the books out on the dining room table and read until the task became daunting. I left the books and went for a bike ride down to the beach to watch the sunset. Soon, I burst into laughter, realizing how silly I was to buy all those books. The doctor had earned my respect. He had more insight into me than I ever imagined. Although not fully convinced of his diagnosis, he seemed so confident, so I decided to trust him.

The next day, I wrapped my impulsive tail between my legs and drove back to the bookstore to return eleven of the thirteen books. The same clerk looked at me with the same smirk.

"It turns out my research project isn't as big as I first anticipated."

"Uh huh."

Within the first four weeks, Ritalin altered my grey matter, but not for the better.

I pleaded with the doctor over the phone, "I have the jitters. I don't know if this is normal, but I can't sit still, and I'm losing weight. I'm already underweight for my height and I can't control my movements. It's as if I'm guzzling shots of espresso."

"That's unfortunate. Some people do react this way, since Ritalin's a stimulant."

"A stimulant? That seems counterproductive."

"We'll have to try something else. I want you to taper off that, and I'll write you a prescription for Wellbutrin."

Wellbutrin only lasted two weeks because it caused me severe dizziness and nausea. It felt like eating a large Mexican plate combo, drinking a few tequila shots, and being strapped in a roller coaster speeding through perilous turns all day.

Next came Prozac. Less exciting than Wellbutrin, but unpleasant in its own way. I suffered from insomnia, endured tension headaches, and felt lethargic like a slug attempting to climb Mt. Kilimanjaro.

I tried a rainbow of Selective Serotonin Reuptake Inhibitors (SSRIs), including Paxil. Nothing helped. The process of taking new medications and tapering off them when they didn't work brought extreme anxiety, replacing depression with a host of symptoms that weren't an improvement. My alter ego name would have been Ms. Edginess. Paranoid, delusional, and OCD in full swing. It even felt like my hair stood at attention, straight out of my head.

After many months, the side effects from all the chemicals flowing in and out of me felt overwhelming. Medication was not my solution, and I doubted I even had ADHD. Although my urgent desire for death had waned, I understood there was still something wrong with me and believed there was another way to fix it.

I thanked the psychiatrist for his help, expressing how much I appreciated the kindness he showed me, but it was time to seek another type of therapy, without drugs. I needed to go deeper, to explore my past that I had suppressed for many years. It was time to bid farewell to Ms. Edginess, find Cherie, and let my hair down.

chapter eleven

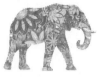

COUNSELING 101

AUGUST 1999 – SAN DIEGO

I drove to meet Brenda, a therapist recommended by my hairdresser. I had nothing to lose but a few hours a week and some hard-earned money.

Brenda was an attractive middle-aged woman of less-than-average height with short dark hair and an impeccable style. Her voice and mannerisms came as soothing as a piano sonata, and her demeanor comforting and calm.

"Cherie, I'm so glad you decided to come in and see me," Brenda said. "Those times we chatted on the phone, I could sense you needed to talk with someone. I'm here to help you."

Her office appeared cozy and sparsely decorated, like a day spa. I sat on a soft leather couch that invited relaxation, and she sat attentive in an ergonomic black chair across from me.

Brenda didn't take notes, only listened while I spent hours answering her questions. Until I met Brenda, I never believed I required counseling, but my opinion soon changed.

The first of my realizations felt the easiest.

"I'm curious," she said. "You say you're a neat and organized person. Have you always been this way?"

"Ever since I can remember." I fidgeted, noticing a wicker trash can with crumpled tissues in it.

She swiveled slightly in her chair. "Let's talk about that. What do you remember about yourself as a young girl, being so neat and concerned with organization?"

Glancing around Brenda's office, I spotted a Tiffany lamp shining on a pile of disheveled papers on her desk and a plant by the window that needed dusting. On the wall behind Brenda, a picture of a butterfly hung crooked. I fought the urge to walk over and straighten it.

"I'm the youngest of three kids. My brother, the oldest, always had his own room. My sister and I shared a room from when I was born until tenth grade. It looked like an episode of the Brady Bunch combined with the Odd Couple. Most times we enjoyed playing games, dressing up in our mother's clothes and putting on makeup.

"Other times we fought and wanted to draw a line down the middle of the room. My sister was disorganized, at least by my unrealistic standards. I couldn't stand to have anything out of place. Everything had to be just so. Her side of the room bothered me, and I bet my side annoyed her. To me, living in a messy room was harmful and chaotic, something I couldn't control, and I—"

Brenda nodded. "So you felt anxious?"

"Yeah, I guess I never thought of it that way. Both my brother and sister were confident, strong, and intelligent. I looked up to them, and loved them so much. I wanted them, and my parents, to love me and think I was good. I was a skinny girl with a meek personality. My brother and sister used to tease me, tricked me into eating dog food, and even once told me I was adopted. Normal sibling stuff. I got teased in school a lot too. They called me Chicken Legs and Cherry Pie. The older kids always asked if I still had my cherry. I didn't know what it meant until later, but was embarrassed just the same. In third grade, some boys came up behind me on the playground during recess and pulled down my sundress, exposing my bare chest. They told everyone I had no breasts. I cried and hid in the bathroom for the rest of the day. I didn't dare wear a strapless dress again until high school. I know all kids go through that kind of stuff. I probably had it easy."

She clasped her hands together in her lap. "I wouldn't say that was easy, but yes, most kids do experience something like what you've described. Still, it doesn't explain why you were so anxious. Can you recall what prompted your anxiety?"

"I do remember feeling the constant need to prove myself to everyone. I tried to be the good girl and do everything right, so they would love me. I suppose that would explain my bedding ritual."

"Bedding ritual?"

"As a young girl, I took great care getting in and out of bed. At bedtime, I removed each one of my fifty or so stuffed animals and placed them neatly on the floor next to my bed. Next, I pulled back my bedspread, only exposing a tiny corner, and climbed up onto the bed at the top next to the wall before I slid underneath the blanket and sheets, trying not to move them out of place.

"I pulled the top cover tightly under my neck, stretched out my left arm, and tucked my hand between the bedding and the wall, making sure it was tight, then stretched my right arm out to the other side and tucked my right hand into the fold of the mattress and the box spring. I stayed stiff as a corpse, my hands tucked in, and my legs together.

"I always woke in the same position, the covers all neatly in place. I un-tucked my hands and slid out of the covers to the top of the bed and stepped down to the floor. The bed looked like it had never been slept in. I put each stuffed animal back in place every day. As I grew older, the habit faded, but it took years to stop it completely."

She gave me a compassionate look. "Cherie, it seems like you had a lot of anxiety and insecurity as a child. You desperately wanted your own space, to be your own person."

I repositioned myself on the couch and studied Brenda. My energy shifted as if a window had opened. By being aware of my anxiety, I became more at ease with it.

Brenda flashed a reassuring smile. "It seems like you were tentative and didn't have a sturdy voice. To cope with your insecurity, you found ways to control the things you could, like keeping your belongings tidy. You even controlled the way you slept, because you could."

My shoulders relaxed. "That makes so much sense. I remember when I went to any of my friends' houses to play, I never accepted food or drinks, or used the bathroom. I didn't want to bother anyone or cause any sort of inconvenience."

She nodded. "It sounds like you were trying to be invisible. By being neat, attentive, and always the good girl who did her chores and homework on time, you were doing what you thought was necessary to get what you craved and what every child wants—love."

I hesitated, feeling an ache deep in my heart for the young me. "What's interesting is I moved out of my parents' house when I was eighteen and went away to college. I love my family. My parents gave me a wonderful childhood. They worked hard to give us everything we needed and were both caring and devoted to us kids. However, I could hardly wait to be on my own, to explore the world. To be free."

She leaned back in her chair and crossed her legs. "And to explore yourself. Remember, you spent your childhood trying to be someone you thought your family, and everyone else in your life, wanted you to be. You probably didn't realize it then, but you couldn't wait to just be yourself."

I felt the truth in her words. It felt like stepping off an airplane knowing that soon I would be home. I always tried to please everyone. I wanted them to like me, so I molded myself into what I thought other people wanted me to do, say, or be.

"Do you have any family in San Diego?" Brenda added.

"No. But I love it here and have so many wonderful friends. It feels like home to me."

"You do seem right at home here. And friends can often be as close, if not closer, than family."

I nodded. Through the window in her office, I saw the sunlight on the palm trees in the distance and felt fortunate to live in San Diego, to know Brenda. I felt a new burst of hope.

chapter twelve

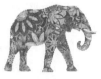

OPENING UP

JANUARY 2000 – SAN DIEGO

After seeing Brenda for months, my feelings of despair lessened, but a final breakthrough lay ahead, the most complicated and arduous of all.

I opened up to Brenda in a way I had never done before with anyone else, with no agenda, no need for validation, sympathy, or a particular reaction. Week after week I unveiled the being inside my thoughts, inside my childhood, formative years, and early adulthood.

She observed that I glossed over parts of my past and treated them as if they were normal and unworthy of attention, until she noticed my facade of strength.

I reclined on the leather couch and stared out the window of Brenda's office. Birds swooped from tree to tree, confused clouds floated by. I wondered what it would feel like to fly. I envisioned my body weightless, soaring.

The softness of Brenda's voice brought me back to the moment. "Cherie, it's not healthy to push all of those feelings down inside of you."

"I'm fine with everything that happened to me in Zambia, really."

"From what I've heard, you seem to understand the magnitude of what occurred, although I still think you're unknowingly diminishing your experience a bit."

"Many people have gone through far worse than I did."

She leaned forward. "That may be true, but we aren't talking about other people, we're talking about you. It isn't even your time in Africa I'm most concerned with. You've withstood other significant traumas you haven't addressed, specifically that incident while you were a college student, before Africa. You alluded to it and moved on quickly."

I stood and walked to the window, watching the birds. "I don't know what to tell you. There isn't much I can do about it, and I'm fine. Really, I'm fine."

"My point exactly. I think for a long time you've told yourself you're fine with all that happened, but you're not fine. You have coped for so long by pushing yourself forward from one activity to another. This is the first time you've ever stopped to take a breath and examine your past. Your subconscious is bringing your past traumas to the surface so you can face them and work through them to clear your depression and anger toward yourself. You need to open up and enable yourself to experience those suppressed feelings."

It wasn't until Brenda pointed it out that I understood how much I downplayed what I had endured. Why did I feel so compelled to pretend it didn't bother me?

I turned and faced Brenda. Her tone came caring and reassuring. "I think it would help you, when you're ready, to talk about it in more detail. Only when you're ready."

Would I be able to let down my guard and not just tell the story, but really feel it?

A week passed. Brenda closed her office door, sat across from me, and smiled. "You look like you have something on your mind."

"I'd like to talk about the incident," I said, feeling an uneasiness rise within me.

"I'm so glad you feel ready. This is going to help you a lot. Say as little or as much as you need. And here, just in case," she handed me a box of tissues with daisies printed on the sides. Daises were my favorite flower. So simple. So unassuming.

"Thank you." I cleared my throat, nervous and scared of what might unravel. "I don't understand why it suddenly feels difficult. It's not as if I haven't told this to anyone before. I guess this time feels different, as if I'm about to relive it."

"Don't think too much about it. Let's just see where this goes, and, Cherie, take your time."

I settled onto the couch and thought back to May 1992. I had recently turned twenty-one and returned from my junior year abroad studying at the University of Hull, in northern England, back to San Diego....

"Welcome home." Alister wrapped his arms around me. His hair light brown and curly, his eyes hazel, just as I remembered.

"Hey, you." I hugged him back. He smelled like soap and hair gel. I missed his scent, his deep voice, his hugs, even his silly goatee.

I yelled to my two roommates, "I'll see you later." I stepped outside, and closed the door to my apartment. The setting sun rested on the apartment building, and the salty ocean air from the nearby beach felt soothing.

He pointed to his truck parked down the street from my apartment. "How's it feel to be back in San Diego?"

I followed him. "It's only been a few days, so I'm still not used to it, but what I love most about being back is the sunshine. For the year I was gone, I felt like I only saw the sun twice in that gloomy little fishing port."

"No wonder you all drink so much."

"What am I, British now?" I giggled.

"Hardly, but from what you've told me in your letters, you learned to drink like them."

"I lived like the locals, absorbed the culture." I chuckled. "Most of the other students at the university drank far more than I did. Plus at nights, it was part of my job."

"I didn't know working as a barmaid in a pub meant you needed to drink, only that you had to serve it."

"Funny." Being with him always made me smile. "I told you about my boss and how he always said, 'long as you can still do your job and you're not too sloshed, you can drink as much as you like.' And besides, it would've been rude not to accept all of those drinks the locals gave me as tips."

Alister smiled, unlocked his truck and opened the passenger door. "It's good to see you, Cherie."

"You too, Alister." I climbed in. "Where we going?"

"To drink, of course," he laughed and closed the door.

He drove south on the freeway while I looked out the window at passing cars, feeling strange on the right side of the road. I glanced at Alister. His eyes focused ahead, unaware of my gaze or thoughts about our relationship. We had only dated for the summer before I left to live in England, but I cared for him. We had agreed to keep an open relationship during my time abroad, and when I returned we would see how we felt. I wanted to be with him again.

He drove us to a hole-in-the-wall bar located on the outskirts of a lively beach town called Pacific Beach. There was no parking on the busy street, which hosted close to fifty bars and restaurants over the span of two miles. This town had a spirited nightlife and was popular with college students.

Wednesday night. The streets were not as crowded as on the weekends, but parking was always at a premium. Alister parked a couple of blocks away, and we walked over to a bar.

Its outside looked unremarkable and barely visible to cars or pedestrians except for a golden sign with faded off-white lights that flashed, *The Gold Mine*. The inside looked narrow, dark, and sparsely decorated with sports paraphernalia, a jukebox, and a dartboard. One television hung on the wall next to the bar. Two small pool tables sat in a corner and a half dozen bar stools filled the rest of the room. It smelled like cigarettes and peanuts. There were only a few people inside, including the bartender and a bored waitress.

Alister and I sat at the bar and ordered beers. The easygoing bartender gave us a couple rounds of vodka shots for free, making us tipsy.

"I'm glad you're back," Alister said while peeling the label off his beer bottle.

"I've missed everything here. I've missed you," I said, anxious for his reply.

"I've missed you too. I care about you, Cherie." His voice cracked. He wiped a bead of sweat from his brow.

My heart skipped.

"But," he hesitated, "I've been seeing someone." He stared at the beer in his hands, unable to look at me.

"That's great," I lied. I too looked at my beer and took a swig, hoping to feel soothed, but felt only emptiness, like I had been punched in the gut.

"Yeah, she's great. I mean, you are too, of course, but I'm involved with her, and I want to continue to see her. I'm hoping you and I can still be friends."

"Of course." I wondered what this girl had that I didn't. "I wasn't sure what to expect when I saw you. We never wrote about our love lives in our letters." I swallowed a large amount of beer. "I'm glad you're happy."

"Thanks for understanding. I don't want to lose you as a friend."

I had dated while I was overseas, but once I got back to San Diego, I wanted to see where things would go with Alister. How had I not seen this coming? I motioned to the bartender for one more vodka shot and swished it back. By this time, I had two beers and two shots swimming in my stomach. A year earlier, I would have been passed out on the floor, but because of the drinking stamina I had developed in Britain, I was inebriated, but lucid enough to function.

Alister went to the jukebox and selected a handful of songs. We played a couple of rounds of pool and reminisced about old times. I tried to keep my composure, laughing and joking, but my hurt feelings magnified as the night progressed. I didn't want to just be his friend. I wanted to leave. I couldn't look at him anymore.

He told me stories of his job and some trips he had taken. I listened, but inside I felt consumed with damaged pride. I longed to run away.

We spent another couple of hours talking. He had stopped drinking since he was driving. I continued my misery-hiding consumption with the cooperation of the overly eager barkeep.

"It's getting late, you ready to go home?" Alister put his hand on my shoulder. I reveled in his touch. I wanted more.

"Yu-up," I slurred, trying to compose myself.

"Wait here, and I'll go get the truck," Alister said as he paid the bartender for the last round of drinks. "I'll just be a few minutes. Wait here, okay?"

I nodded and watched him leave.

A minute later, I hopped off the barstool, thanked the bartender for the great service, and wandered out the front door into the night. I looked right and left, but Alister was nowhere in sight. I figured it would be at least five minutes before he returned, and I didn't want to be there when he did. I couldn't bear to look at him anymore knowing he was in love with someone else.

Turning left down the sidewalk, I headed toward the more populated part of the town to hail a cab, go home, and cry myself to sleep. It hadn't occurred to me that I was back in San Diego and taxis were not sitting in front of bars waiting to take people home like in England.

I walked steadfast and forward, pulling my cardigan around my chest. My eyelids fluttered, and my eyes strained to focus through my inebriation. Ten steps forward and a deep voice called my name. I turned around, expecting Alister, but didn't see him, or anyone else. I turned back around and continued a few more steps. Once again I heard a robust voice say, "Cherie." I glimpsed a tan face, blond hair, and white T shirt coming toward me.

I saw an arm and felt something hard hit the back of my skull, then black.

I woke up with a throbbing headache. My vision was blurry and I fought to concentrate.

What happened? Where am I?

I wasn't standing. I was lying down with an uneven surface of jagged and cold gravel beneath me. My head faced up, my vision tuned into the dark night sky and a couple of faint stars. My head pounded, and the cool night air rushed along my legs. My arms felt stiff and restrained.

My eyes opened, and the man in the white T-shirt, whom I did not recognize but who knew my name, was on top of me, moving, grunting.

My black skirt was up around my waist, and my black cotton underwear stretched and pushed to the left of my upper thigh. This stranger was inside me. He had pinned me down with his arms and was rocking back and forth on top of me.

"No!" I shouted, "No!"

I sank heavy like lead into the rough ground below me and shook my head violently, yelling "Help me!" while kicking my legs and trying to free my arms from his grasp.

He was too strong.

My screams for help reached no one. I saw nothing but an aged chain-link fence surrounding the abandoned parking lot I was in. Before I could take another breath and scream again for help, the stranger hit me over the head and again, nothing.

chapter thirteen

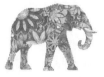

DARKNESS TO DAWN

JANUARY 2000 – SAN DIEGO

My attention shifted back to Brenda's office, the taupe walls, the Tiffany lamp on the desk, the soft sunken couch supporting my sluggish body, and Brenda's face lit with concern.

"Are you okay?" Brenda probed.

Tears welled up in my eyes.

"I'm so upset I was drinking. If I hadn't been drunk, I might have waited for Alister, and it wouldn't have happened. I wasn't thinking clearly." I felt flustered and shook.

"Cherie, we as women should be able to walk down a city street, hail a cab, and feel safe. You were not doing anything wrong. He attacked you."

"I know, but—"

"There are no buts. He attacked and raped you. Whether you were drinking or not, it was not your fault. You need to know that."

"That's what I try to tell myself, but I still feel—"

"Cherie. Stop. What happened is not your fault. Do you hear what I'm saying?"

"Yes. But it's difficult to absorb. I put myself in danger by drinking that much and walking out of that bar."

"Drinking, even in excess, is in no way responsible for what happened to you."

"You're right," I muttered, drying my eyes with a scrunched tissue.

"What he did to you was horrible. I think you're inappropriately blaming yourself. Your anger should be toward this man for what he did to you."

"I am angry. So angry someone would do something like that to me, or to anyone. I hate that I can't feel safe walking alone without fear of being attacked." My indignation escalated. My voice rose. "I'm maddened he violated my body and took something private from me, and I had no chance to do anything to stop it."

"You have every right to be angry. He hurt you. Even though this was years ago, it seems you've never allowed yourself to feel these emotions." Brenda gave me a nurturing gaze.

"I don't think I ever got angry before," I said.

"Let it out."

"I'm angry!" I yelled. "I hate what he did to me. I hate it!" I sobbed, took a tissue from the box, and wiped my eyes.

Brenda studied me for a couple of minutes while I cried before she spoke. "Is there anything else you feel besides anger?"

"I feel disgusting. I'm repulsed with my body and what he did to it." My anger swelled. "It isn't right!"

"I know. You went through a traumatic experience, something not easy to accept and live with, especially since you've carried it around for so long."

"What scares me still is that he knew my name. I remember feeling crazed by this detail. He may have known me." I took a deep breath.

"This man probably overheard your name in the bar and followed you as you left. The odds are he didn't know you before that night."

"That could be true, but for a long time after that, anywhere I went, I believed he could be watching me, waiting to attack me again. I felt naked, and still do in a sense, because I will never know who he is, or where he is. The worst part is there's more."

"Do you want to continue, or would you rather talk about the rest next session?"

"I want to finish now if we have enough time."

"Plenty. Go ahead." Brenda sat back in her chair and rested her chin on her hand, listening.

"This next part I don't remember. I was told later that two police officers found me passed out and propped up against a dumpster in the empty lot. The perpetrator, or someone else, stole my purse. With no identification and smelling of alcohol, the police took me to a detoxification facility in downtown San Diego and left me there to sleep and recover. I don't think they had any idea I had been raped."

I grabbed a tissue, blew my nose, and proceeded to drink the last of the water in my paper cup. Brenda took my cup and refilled it. I recalled the rest of that night....

I woke in the detox center on a thin, lumpy mattress between two tall gray partitions that separated me from the rest of what looked like an old warehouse.

My thoughts felt congested. I didn't know where I was or where I had been. My senses worked to ascertain information. Faint background music came from a small radio, a Mexican station. I smelled sweat and cheap cologne. My hands and feet felt cold, and the taste of stale beer filled my mouth.

Still foggy from alcohol, I opened my eyes. My head throbbed, and I sensed something was wrong.

Before I could collect my thoughts, I felt deplorable sensations in the most sensitive parts of me. I looked down and couldn't believe what I saw and felt. A sizable man, olive-skinned with dark flowing hair, and thick black glasses, hovered over me, his hand up inside me, molesting me.

I could hardly breathe. I pushed away from him, kicking and shouting. Startled, he jumped backwards. I sprang to my feet and ran through a labyrinth of partitions and mattresses, not knowing where I was, or where I needed to go. I found a front entrance and ran past an unattended desk with the radio playing music. I moved fast, pulling my skirt down, then pushed the glass door of the detox center open and darted out into unfamiliar city streets.

I sprinted down the street, never looking behind me. My head ached, yet I felt sober and cruelly aware.

High-rises and tall apartment buildings loomed over me like brown and gray monsters, guffawing as I fled. I ran faster. On top of one of these aberrations, a large clock with black iron edging showed 3 a.m.

I need a taxi. Please, where is a taxi?

Across the street, on an empty street corner in front of a nightclub with a neon pink sign, I glimpsed a green and white car. I ran toward it, grabbed the door handle, tumbled into the back seat, and closed the door, panting.

"Where to?" the cabbie said.

"Solana Beach."

He turned on the meter and drove off to my apartment close to thirty-five miles away.

We traveled far above the speed limit in the fast lane on the freeway. I shook my head, haunted by that strange man's face and what he had done to me. I glanced down at my legs. Iridescent dried trails of something covered my thighs. I rubbed my hand against my legs and up toward my waist, feeling a thick, crusty substance. A horrible twinge shot through me when I sensed the same matter between my legs, lining my underwear.

I saw flashbacks of the other man with the blond hair, yelling my name, knocking me out, waking up, and him moaning and inside of me. I shut my eyes and sank deep into the seat and cried.

The driver peered at me through the rear-view mirror. I pushed my legs tight together and looked away, gazing out the window, wondering what the driver thought. Did he know? Could he smell the rape, or see the dried semen on my legs? Could he tell from my disheveled appearance, or did he see it on my face as I unraveled the events of the night in my mind? A broken heart from a man I once loved, and a broken body and spirit from two disparate strangers—all in one horrible night. I couldn't wait to get home, take a shower, and cleanse the filth invading my skin.

The cabbie pulled up in front of my apartment.

"I'll be right back."

I sprinted up the stairs to my apartment, rang the doorbell, and pounded on the door. My roommates, Jill and Elise, answered. I begged them to lend me some money. They pooled their cash, and I paid the driver.

I rushed back inside, closed and locked the door behind me, and collapsed on the living room floor.

"What's wrong, Cherie? What happened?" Jill asked.

My arms and legs shook. I blurted out bits and pieces from my scattered thoughts.

Elise held me close while Jill called the police.

"The police said we should take you to the hospital to see a doctor and give a full report." Jill placed the phone on the table.

"I have to shower first. I feel so dirty." I tried to stand.

Jill's voice came soft. "No. You have to wait until after they examine you. It's important. I'm sorry."

I wailed.

Elise hugged me and said, "Come on, we need to get you to the hospital. I'll drive."

At a hospital in La Jolla, Jill and Elise sat in the waiting room as a nurse escorted me into a private, well-lit room that had one exam table and a row of curtains hanging from the ceiling, and smelled of sanitizer.

I stood naked in the middle of the room while a young Japanese-American woman doctor named Dr. Delicate and the nurse scoured my body for evidence. They plucked pubic hairs, took samples from my thighs and in between my legs, and conducted a full pelvic examination. A soft tap on the door brought a female police officer named Officer Compassionate who asked questions and snapped photographs while the other two continued their inspections.

It was difficult enough having anyone poke and prod me after what I had been through. Thankfully, all three were female.

Humiliated and overwhelmed, I shook through the entire examination and questioning. I wanted to curl up in a little ball of flesh and float away, but they needed to do their job, especially if they had any hope of catching those men.

Officer Compassionate took detailed notes and asked a multitude of questions. I recounted the entire night, relaying as many details as I could, as I lay with my legs spread up in stirrups and my shivering skin covered only by a stiff, thin white paper gown.

After the doctor finished scraping samples from my underwear, the officer asked if she could take it as evidence. I nodded. My head throbbed, some from the head injury, some from the alcohol, and some from the trauma.

The examination and questioning felt like days, but it had only been two hours.

"Okay, Cherie, we're done," said Dr. Delicate.

I watched the doctor and police officer leave the room.

"There's a bathroom with a shower at the end of the hall. Here are the clothes your roommates brought for you." The nurse paused then said, "I'm sorry this happened to you."

People passed me as I walked through the hallway. I clung to my gown. Did everyone in the hospital know why I was there?

I stepped into the bathroom, locked the door, dropped my gown, and hurried into the shower. The knob on the shower moved easily. Scalding water pressed against my chest while I scrubbed my skin, washing away the perpetrators' filthy scents, the despicable traces they left on me, and in me. I couldn't scrub hard enough. My flesh looked reddened and raw. I had to stop before my skin bled.

Dressed, I headed toward the waiting room. Officer Compassionate stopped me and handed me her business card.

"If you think of anything else, please call me. Otherwise, I'll be in touch. Take care."

Seconds after she left, Dr. Delicate approached me from the other side of the hall.

"Cherie, I'll let you know about those tests we ran, but I advise you to repeat them with your regular doctor." She handed me a slip of paper, my discharge instructions. "Do them every six months for a while to be sure."

I nodded, realizing the threat from that night wasn't over. Could I have contracted some sort of STD from the man who raped me? HIV?

No, I can't think that way.

The doctor placed a hand on my shoulder and gestured toward the exit. With my head down, I pushed open the door, signaled to my friends, and walked into the dawn.

chapter fourteen

LUCKY ME

JANUARY 2000 – SAN DIEGO

Sunlight sparkled in through Brenda's office window near the couch where I sat. A row of dust motes danced in the air, and I tried to take a deep breath, but it was shallow.

"I'm sorry for everything you went through." Brenda reached out her hand to me. "Are you doing okay?"

"I'm exhausted. Can we finish next time?"

"Of course. If you need me for anything before then, just call."

During the week between sessions, I focused on that night, every sight, scent, noise, and feeling. A waterfall of emotions poured out of me, leaving me empty in a beautiful way.

The next week I arrived at Brenda's office feeling relieved and a little lighter.

"Before you conclude your story, Cherie, how are you doing?"

"I'm doing well, considering. Last session was difficult, and all week my thoughts kept bringing me back to that time, but I feel I'm dealing with it better than I did back when it all happened. I remember the next day feeling so exposed. I didn't want anyone to see me like that, and honestly, I didn't know quite how to deal with everything that had happened." I stretched out on Brenda's couch and resumed my story....

I woke at noon the day after the attack. I felt groggy and my skull throbbed, as if someone had used my head as a bass drum. I stumbled downstairs, sat at the table, and stared at the kitchen appliances. Both famished and parched, I grabbed a glass of water and fought to shake the memories of the previous night. It was not a nightmare. It was dreadful, and it was real.

I stood in the center of our kitchen staring at a poster that hung over our dining room table of a surfer riding a wave. He looked exhilarated and peaceful.

"Cherie, Alister's on the phone," Elise called out. "Do you want to talk with him?"

I hadn't heard the phone ring. I took the receiver from her. "Hello," I whispered.

"Hey. I'm glad you're all right. I went back to the bar to pick you up and I couldn't find you anywhere. The bartender said you left. I figured you were mad at me."

"I'm not mad at you. And don't worry, I'm home. I'm fine." I started sobbing.

"What's going on?"

"I...I..."

"Do you want me to come over?"

"No."

"What's going on?"

"Please, leave me alone."

"But, Cherie—"

"I'm fine."

"You don't sound fine. I'll come over, we can talk about it."

"Wait. Don't. I'll tell you." I explained in general terms what had happened and that I was okay, and I didn't need him to do anything.

"Oh God, Cherie. I'm sorry. I'm so sorry. Damn it! I shouldn't have left you!"

"You didn't do anything wrong, Alister. And look," I wiped my tears with my sleeve, "it's over. Okay? I don't want to talk about it."

"I'm coming over. I'll be right there." Alister hung up.

I placed the phone on my lap and lowered my head onto the table. My heart felt as though it was thumping against my rib cage.

Be strong. Don't let him see how much you're hurting. It's nothing. It's no big deal. Tell him what he wants to hear and say goodbye.
That's what I did.

I sunk lower on Brenda's couch. I wiped my eyes and added another used tissue to the pile next to me. "There was no time to sulk. I needed a job. I had to pay rent and buy food. The second day after the attack, I pushed my feelings deep inside me, and started working as a valet at a posh restaurant on the beach, the same job I'd had before I left for England."

Brenda nodded and studied me as I continued my story. "A week after that lurid incident, something prompted me to push that night further down into my subconscious....

I borrowed my roommate's compact, champagne-colored 1967 Chevette hatchback, since my destination was farther than I could cycle, and drove home from doing my errands early afternoon on a Wednesday. The song *Hold on My Heart* by Phil Collins played on the stereo. The melody felt soothing, filling me with the first sensation of joy I had experienced since the attack. The rhythm cradled my fragile soul and gave me a spark of hope that I would one day feel comfortable in my own skin.

The sky appeared cloudless and the faintest of blues. The cliffs beside me, craggy and brown, topped with Torrey pine trees. I drove down the Pacific Coast Highway from the UCSD campus to the pristine, dark-blue ocean water at the bottom of the hill, the two lanes merged into one. I looked and saw no one on the road, then looked in the rear-view mirror. No one behind me.

I sang along to the chorus, trying to decipher the lyrics, looking ahead. In an instant, from the beach parking lot on my left, a maroon four-door luxury car pulled in front of me.

I had two choices: veer to the right and drive over the edge of the street into the lagoon and marsh, or slam on the brakes and hope and pray I didn't hit him.

I choose option two.

The brakes locked. I slammed into him at forty-five miles an hour.

The big car flew off into the marsh, and the Chevette did a 180, ending up on the median dividing the two opposing lanes. My forehead, knees, and arms bashed into the steering wheel. I was wearing my seat belt, but it was old and slack, and didn't fully protect me.

Once the car stopped, I felt my head thumping. I looked in the tilted mirror dangling from the windshield. My forehead swelled. My knees were jammed up against the steering wheel, and I was shaking. The muscles around my neck, head, and shoulders tightened. It felt like time had stopped. I heard my breathing, felt my pulse increase, and smelled blood on my face.

A man ran up to the driver's side of my car. "Miss, you okay?"

I tried to shake my head but couldn't. My chest and legs were crushed up against the steering wheel.

"I called 911. The ambulance is on its way," the stranger said in a calm voice.

"It's not my car. She's going to be so mad," I muttered.

"Look miss, I saw the whole thing. That guy cut you off. It was his fault not yours, don't worry."

The ambulance arrived. Two paramedics approached. The driver door was dented in and the car looked like an accordion in the middle of playing a tune. They pried the door open, lifted me out of the vehicle, and placed me on a stretcher.

The witness stood close by as the paramedics raised me into the van. He reiterated, "Don't worry. I'll wait for the police and call the hospital with the information from the other driver."

The doors closed. I looked up at the paramedic nearest to me, his face white and his hair black. He examined me and said, "From the looks of that accident, if you weren't wearing your seat belt you might not have made it."

"But—"

"Try not to speak. I know, the seat belt was loose, but it saved you from being thrown out of the vehicle onto the pavement. We could be taking you to the morgue instead. Be thankful for that."

Lying on the stretcher in the same hospital in La Jolla where I had endured the rape exam, I waited for the doctor. I remembered one of the last things I had seen before I hit the steering wheel—the car in front of me had two people in the front seat, and a white New York license plate that read "The Empire State."

The doctor, Dr. Blurry, who wore thick glasses that rivaled Martin Scorsese's, pointed to my forehead. "Ms. Kephart, you have a skull-line fracture across here." He held up a small mirror so I could see. My forehead protruded over my eyes. I looked like a Neanderthal.

"You also have severe whiplash in your neck. That's why you can't move your head. You're going to need to wear this." Dr. Blurry secured a brace around my neck.

The muscles in my neck felt like rigid metal cables. I fought the urge to scream. "For how long?"

"I'm not sure, depends on how well you recover from this. Surprisingly, the X-rays came back fine. You had quite the accident."

"What about my arms and knees?" Bruises had formed on all of them.

Dr. Blurry looked me over. "There doesn't seem to be any internal damage, just some contusions. I'm going to recommend extensive physical therapy for at least six months, maybe longer."

I couldn't move my head, and it ached to walk because my knees refused to bend properly. This latest trauma overshadowed the rape and molestation.

I called my roommates and shared what had happened. I was so grateful they were there for me and could come pick me up. While I waited, the witness from the beach called the hospital.

"I wanted to let you know I stayed and told the police everything."

"What about the people in the other car. Are they all right?" I asked.

"They're fine. They got out and walked away without a scratch. I made certain they gave me and the police all of their information. They have insurance, so that should take care of everything."

"Thank you. You're so kind." I felt moved by his willingness to help me.

"You're welcome. I gave my information to the police, so if you need me to testify or anything, I'll be happy to."

"Again, thanks." I felt a small portion of my faith in unknown men restored.

Brenda gave me a caring look. I sat up on the couch, took a sip of water, and glanced at her, thankful she was a female, since I doubted I could confide in a man.

"This explains why you didn't deal with the attack. You didn't have the opportunity to," Brenda said.

"It became more difficult because although my roommate Jill was concerned with my well-being, as days passed I could see how displeased she was about her car. She said it wasn't my fault, but her unhappiness toward me became evident.

"I don't know how I could have avoided the accident. I assured her that somehow I would pay for her car if the other driver's insurance didn't. Unfortunately, my accident ruined our friendship. Since I was disabled and in physical therapy five days a week for the entire summer, I couldn't work. I had to move out because I couldn't afford the rent. I moved to a cheaper place closer to physical therapy and university so I could take the bus. I couldn't cycle that far."

"This is important." Brenda shifted in her chair and sat up straighter. "You suffered such a dreadful accident that your physical wounds overrode your emotional scars from the week before. Your attention was focused on healing and getting back to work so you could pay your bills. This forced you to push aside the attack. And, if I'm correct, you probably never dealt with it much again."

I instinctively rubbed my neck. "I was in physical therapy for close to a year. I wore a neck brace for almost a month, and I had to go back to work sooner than my doctor wanted because I was broke. Needing money, healing my injuries, and paying back my roommate took precedence.

"Because of that witness, it was proven the other driver was at fault. All my medical bills and my roommate's car were eventually paid in full, but it took a year to settle the case and get the money from the insurance company. Until that time, I struggled to pay my bills. I worked full-time while completing my senior year in college. The good news is I paid everything off, and I graduated the following spring on time."

"What ever happened with the investigation from the police about that night?" Brenda asked.

"Oh, yeah. Two days after the car accident, the investigating police officer for my sexual assault case came by to visit me...."

"Hello, officer, please come in." I closed my apartment door behind us, limped through the living room, and sat at the dining room table beneath the surfing poster. Officer Compassionate sat next to me and placed a large white envelope on the table. She wore police-issued sunglasses and a pant suit, and smelled like she'd had garlic for lunch.

"Cherie, what happened? That brace and your head isn't from the incident?" She removed her sunglasses and stared at me. I tried to cover some of my bruising with my hair.

"Believe it or not, I got in a car accident. This guy pulled in front of me. Not a great outcome."

"I'm so sorry. You've had such a horrible week."

"You could say that."

"The reason I'm here is because I wanted to let you know our lab tests confirmed semen on your underwear."

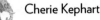

"Oh gosh," I whispered, covering my mouth with my hands.

"However, I'm sorry to say there were no matches found."

A trace of stomach acid rose into my throat. I slid my hands up over my eyes.

"I know this is difficult, Cherie, but can you remember anything else about that guy?"

I shook my head. "It's all so hazy." I moved my hands down onto my lap. "I remember the plain white T-shirt, blond hair, and tanned face. He was taller than me, about six feet."

"Unfortunately, that could be more than half of the men in Southern California."

"I know. Isn't there anything else we can do?"

"I'm afraid not. There's little chance we will ever be able to find him. I'm sorry."

How could this be? Where is the justice?

"There is something we might be able to do about the other guy." Officer Compassionate reached into the envelope on the table.

"You mean the second guy, the one at the detox center?"

"We thought maybe he worked there, so we got photographs of all the employees. We hope you'll be able to identify him."

I pointed to the upside-down stack she had in her hand. "Those are the photos?"

She turned over a stack of head shots, all of men, and my heart beat faster as she flipped through them one by one. I shook my head at each new picture until, about halfway through the stack, I gasped. "That's him." A grotesque pang gripped my stomach. Unlike the vision of the faceless rapist I had etched in my mind, this man's face was unmistakable.

"Are you certain?"

"Absolutely. That's him." Even if I wanted to, I could never forget.

Days later Officer Compassionate called me. "Cherie, we went down to the detox center and arrested the man you identified."

I trembled. "You did?"

"Yes. He confessed. He also admitted to molesting several other women over the years that were passed out and unaware. You were the first to wake up during his assault."

"Oh no." That awful night flooded my mind. I recoiled and tried not to think of it.

"Because of your positive I.D., he'll probably be sentenced to six months in prison and a minimum eighteen months of probation after his jail time. Look, he can't hurt you now and he can no longer take advantage of other women."

"I'm glad he can't harm anyone else." My relief felt small.

"Cherie, he gave me a message for you."

I tried to speak, but no words came.

"He told me to tell you he was sorry, and that he had a problem and he didn't mean to hurt you."

But he did.

I couldn't reconcile what to do with his apology. "Will he get help?"

"I hope so."

Brenda looked as if she had something to say. She waited as I composed myself. I sipped some water. Blew my nose. Wiped my tears.

"How do you feel about what he said to you?"

I shook my head. "I still don't know what to do with his apology."

"He had a serious problem, but there's no apology that could ever make right what he did to you. Perhaps over time you can forgive him."

"I feel sad for him. He does have a problem. I just hope he never abuses anyone ever again."

"You said you never told anyone in your family what happened. Why not? Perhaps they could have been there for you."

"I felt ashamed and scared. By the time I thought about confiding in anyone, the car accident happened, which I did tell them about in the same phone call that my mother told me polyps were found in my sister's colon, and she needed to start radiation therapy. She was only twenty-three, two years older than me. My mother sounded terrified about her condition, so I downplayed the accident and decided not to tell her about the rape and molestation."

"Was your sister okay?"

"Yes. She's recovered and is doing great."

Brenda leaned forward. "Can you see how much you went through, and how tough it was for you not being able to share or deal with all that happened to you?"

"To think about all of it strung together is powerful. Something I never talk about is that for years following the attack, I had HIV tests every six months to ensure I hadn't contracted anything. Each test felt terrifying, and waiting for the results—unbearable." I cringed remembering that feeling.

"I hated the thought that the attack could cause me to contract a disease. I'm so grateful that never happened, but I was also scared of being attacked again. I didn't drink for over a year. Even later, once I allowed myself, I only did so moderately and when surrounded by close friends. I'm still a bit frightened to let myself relax."

"You were vulnerable when those men took advantage of you, but you're a strong and brave woman. You've braved things no one should have to. I'm here to talk any time you need to."

"Thank you. I thought I had dealt with it, that I was resilient, but I was a victim. I never wanted to see myself that way, but I was. I suppose we all are victims at some point in our lives. Whenever I think about that night, I realize how lucky I am."

"How so?"

"So many women are raped then murdered. All those men wanted from me was sexual gratification. Either one of them could have killed me. I'm lucky I survived."

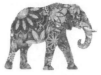

chapter fifteen

DO YOU SMELL SOMETHING?

APRIL 2004, PART III – SAN DIEGO

The morning sun's rays peeked through the window into my bed-room on the day after my visit to the ER with Alex. I felt thankful to have survived the night.

My room smelled musty, the air cool from the breeze flowing in through the cat door. I peered out the window into the backyard and saw both my cats lying in the grass.

I turned on my other side and faced Alex, wincing from pain. All my neck muscles felt like rubber bands stretched and pulled taut as if they were about to snap. "You awake?"

Alex half opened his eyes. "Huh, yeah, hon. You feeling better?"

"Worse."

"I'll get you some water."

"Thank you. I need to call my boss and tell her what's going on." I loved working as a technical writer. It was challenging, and my colleagues were great.

He yawned. "You want me to call her for you and tell her you'll call after the neurologist appointment on Monday?"

"Yes, that would be great. Thank you. Could you please tell her I'm sorry?"

Alex rolled out of bed and left, returning a minute later with a glass of water. He tilted it up to my mouth so I could drink.

"Don't concern yourself with work right now. Your boss will understand. You need to focus on getting better."

"I'm so scared."

"I'll take the day off from work. Don't worry, I'm not leaving you."

"Oh, Alex. You would do that? Thank you so much!"

My symptoms intensified with each passing hour as if someone behind the curtain of my life were turning a pain dial from "agonizing" to "we don't even make gauges that go this high." Nothing eased my pain.

"Alex, I can't take this anymore."

"You want to go back to the ER?"

"They said they can't help me. I don't know what to do."

"You have to hang on through the weekend."

"I don't know if I can wait that long." I held Alex's hand, our fingers interlaced. "Maybe my friend Sandy can help."

"The homeopathic teacher?"

"Her number's in my cell."

An hour later, Sandy, a vibrant, intelligent woman with a compelling sense of self, sat next to me on the edge of my bed wearing a black sweater and burgundy lipstick. She pushed her short, dark hair out of her striking brown eyes and placed her hand on my shoulder.

"Thanks so much for coming over."

"Of course, Cherie. Now, since I've known you, you've been a healthy, strong, and athletic girl. To see you so powerless without explanation, there must be something going on in your life that caused this."

"You know about my knee?" My voice sounded barely audible.

"You had surgery back in October, right?"

"Exploratory surgery that showed nothing. I've been much worse since the procedure."

"How?"

"My knee's more unstable and my heart rate's faster. I'm nervous. My chest is tight. I have trouble breathing."

"I think something went wrong in that surgery," Sandy said. "What else?"

"I've been at my new job for a few months. It's going well. A little stressful but the people are nice. I'm happy there."

"Still technical writing?"

"Yes."

"What about you and Alex?"

"He's great." I took a breath. "We've only been dating a couple of months and wanted to take things slow, but this health stuff makes everything more intense."

I motioned to Alex. "Can you please tell Sandy about the house, I'm exhausted."

He walked over and sat in a chair next to the bed. "I don't think Cherie wants to admit she's renting from an asshole," he said, "since she loves this place, the cheap rent, and proximity to the beach, but it has tons of problems. I'm certain there are health violations."

Sandy looked around the room. "What's wrong with it?"

"She, just a few weeks ago, found mold in her bathrooms and kitchen. She even found some in her bedroom closet and on some of her clothing. She had a plumber inspect everything and reported it to the landlord, who, by the way, owns close to thirty properties in San Diego. He's worth a lot of money. He never responds to her requests and does nothing about the mold. The toilet had mushrooms growing around the base of it. She thought she might fall through the floor using it, so she had to sit on it gingerly at an angle and keep trimming the mushrooms. It took months for the landlord to fix it. They didn't replace the toilet or the sub-flooring, they just put in a cheap piece of linoleum around it to cover up the problem."

She folded her arms. "I'm not sure about those mushrooms, but mold can be toxic, even fatal."

Alex stroked my hair. "I've read about that."

"Anything else?"

Alex continued, "A main sewage pipeline burst underneath this house just recently. Roots from the tree in the front yard caused the damage. The sewage burst up through the shower and the toilets."

Sandy crinkled her nose. "That's terrible."

"Disgusting. It took hours of scrubbing and cleaning sewage from the two bathrooms and parts of the living room. She called a plumber in the middle of the night, which cost a lot of money. The landlord was upset about it too. The plumber did a patch job to get her through the night, but sewage spilled underneath the house. He said he'd come back and fix all the problems, drain and chemically treat the sewage, but the landlord wouldn't approve the work. Finally his workers came. All they did was remove the tree in the front yard that caused the original problem. They refused to clean up the mess under the house. She's been fighting with the landlord since to get him to clean it up properly."

"There's sewage below us?"

"It's dried up by now, but it's still there. Since then it's rained a lot. It pours out onto the yard and around the house."

"This is no way to live. She needs to move. I'm sure this is related to her illness. The tightness in her chest, her trouble breathing. That could be exposure to the mold. Living here's not helping her."

"She was just about to take legal action with the landlord and look for a new place to live when all this health stuff happened."

I faded in and out of awareness, hearing enough to realize that Sandy and Alex agreed I needed to leave this place right away.

Sandy leaned over me. "Cherie, I'm leaving. Call me if you need anything. Alex will take you to see my colleague Penny tomorrow. She's a chiropractor. I'll call her and tell her to fit you in. I think she can help you."

I smiled, and with my eyes closed said, "Thank you."

On Saturday, Alex drove me to Penny's house, about five miles away. I fought to keep still on a massage table in her living room.

A small green statue of Buddha sat by the front door; vibrant peach and fuchsia drapes hung from her windows. Penny looked like a modern hippie, wearing stylish hemp clothing and beaded bracelets.

My heart raced as she twisted and turned my neck, arms, hips, and back. Each modification overpowered me. Only a squirrel receiving a chiropractic adjustment from King Kong would understand.

At the end of the hour, my symptoms were worse than when she started. Propped up against Alex, I paid and thanked Penny, and then he led me outside.

My legs gave way, and an acute pain shot through me like barbed wire wrapped taut around my muscles. I fell to the ground screaming. Alex lifted me up into his Jeep.

"You can't go back to your place. Doesn't Sandy live down the street from here?"

I nodded.

"I'm taking you there."

Sandy and Alex carried me into her master bedroom and put me on a queen-size bed. Fresh lavender filled the air, and I could hear the faint melody of jazz music playing in the next room. I stared at the ceiling since I couldn't risk moving my neck.

"How you doing?" Alex whispered.

"My chest hurts, and my neck, it's so stiff. My left arm feels numb. What's wrong with me?"

"I don't know, hon."

Hours passed. Sandy and Alex stood by as I sobbed and screamed. Sandy called Paloma, a homeopathic healer, a natural beauty who often wore converse shoes and silver jewelry. She treated her patients like family, and her compassion and caring ways were always a gift.

Sandy, Paloma, and an energetic healer named Will, all leaned over me, touching my arms and legs. Images of Zambia flashed through my mind, when Kyle sat beside me, consoling me as I jerked out of control, but this time I wished for life. I pleaded silently: *Please end this torture. I want to live.*

Tears flooded my eyes, yet I could see Alex watching from the back of the room, head slightly hung. My belly convulsed. I screamed.

The three healers encouraged me to let out everything trapped inside. I had no choice. My body took over. I cried for hours until the tears departed and a hollow sensation consumed me.

"You're in no condition to go anywhere. You can stay here until your appointment on Monday," Sandy said.

I didn't have the energy to answer.

Sandy's oldest son gave up his bedroom for me, a gracious present from a seventeen-year-old boy. Alex put me on the twin bed and curled up next to it on the floor with a blanket and pillow.

Although I had so many cradling me with such care, that night in that room, the isolation of my unceasing intense agony made it difficult to see the presence of others. I thanked them for helping me, and extending such friendship and concern, but I still felt far away from everything but pain.

Sandy, her two boys, and Alex all slept, while I begged for an end to my suffering. I stared into the dark. The only light I could see was the neon green glow from the alarm clock across the room. I watched each number turn, wishing I could make them go faster.

The morning brought me no comfort, nor did the rest of the weekend. I scarcely ate and only had feather-light sleep. I lost weight, my chest muscles constricted, and my vision grew blurry. The slightest light, sound, or smell attacked me. I needed a dark quiet place.

In a fetal position on an oversized couch in the middle of Sandy's living room, I stared between the ceiling and the inside of my eyelids while people moved out the front door and down the hall, to the backyard, to the telephone, and all around me to places I could not go. I had no strength to do anything but feel—the last thing I wanted to do.

Monday came. The neurologist, Dr. Friendly from South Africa, was a slim, soft-spoken, middle-aged man. The exam room was meticulous and comforting like him.

Alex relayed to him my symptoms and vast medical history, including several odd problems. I've never had a broken bone, contracted poison ivy, or needed any dental fillings. I tended to get problems more out of the ordinary, such as sleep paralysis; unpredictable spurts of narcolepsy; the bones in my left shoulder fusing together, requiring surgery to shave the bones to create more room in the joint; and missing an entire layer of gums in my mouth, requiring extensive gum surgery at age sixteen. Just to name a few.

Dr. Friendly conducted a lengthy examination, including several basic neurological tests, which took the better part of two hours. The rest of the time he spent talking with and examining me, which was reassuring. I craved someone to listen and try to help me.

Dr. Friendly sat back in his chair and crossed his legs. "Clinically, you seem stable. From the basic neurological tests I conducted, you show no signs of degeneration of the neurological system, despite your symptoms. I would like you to undergo a sequence of tests, including an MRI of your brain, neck, and back; a lumbar puncture; and multiple blood tests."

"What are you looking for? What do you think you might find?" My voice sounded shaky.

"I don't want to guess. I need to see the results of these tests."

"But you suspect something?" Alex said.

"Your symptoms and your exam do not add up. I don't want to say anything specific that might alarm you because we have no idea until we get these tests back."

"I don't think I can be any more scared than I am right now. Please give me an idea what you're thinking."

"Multiple sclerosis is one. Maybe lupus, but from what I've heard and seen, I doubt you have either. The tests I've ordered will help rule these and other diseases out. It may end up being a process of elimination to determine what's wrong, which can take time...."

"What about her living in Africa? And the malaria? You think this could be from that?"

"I'm not sure. We'll do some additional tests."

"What can we do for her in the meantime?"

"Rest as much as you can," he said to me. "I'll write you a prescription to show your boss since it's obvious you can't work."

"Thank you." I grimaced and held my throbbing neck with my left hand.

"What about her pain?" Alex asked.

"I don't want any pain medication if we don't know what we are treating," I said. "I know this can lead to dependency, and masking of the symptoms."

"In that case, I suggest Aleve or Advil, a warm bath, a heating pad, and again, lots of rest. I know you don't feel like it, but make sure you eat; you're quite skinny."

The doctor left. I put my hands together and attempted to hold my head upright. It swayed like a bowling ball supported by a splintering toothpick. Alex came to my side and gave me a gentle embrace. Although my pain remained, my spirit lifted. This neurologist was approachable, knowledgeable, and dedicated to helping. He was everything I hoped he would be. Now, I needed two things: a diagnosis and a cure.

We returned to Sandy's house teeming with hope and yet wary for what unknown circumstances lurked in the ensuing test results.

Monday night progressed, and so did my stress. Nighttime was not my ally. Something in the dimness of light akin to the darkness inside me heightened my fear. Was it my mind playing tricks on me, or was it an unseen set of biological factors contributing to the magnified sense of agony in the night hours?

Alex traveled from his office, to his apartment, to my house (checking on and tending to my two cats), and cared for me at Sandy's home. He brought me food, clothes, and supplies; helped me bathe; and took me to get my MRIs, X-rays, and other tests. His aid was invaluable, his efforts unwavering. Never did he ask what was in it for him.

Days passed and blended into each other. By Friday I had been at Sandy's home a week. She placed a portable stereo next to me on the floor. I tossed and turned on the couch in her living room, staring at her lush garden outside the window and listening to CDs of soothing-ocean and flowing-brook sounds in an attempt to distract myself, but all they did was make me want to pee.

Sandy opened up her home to me in one of my most desperate times, but my condition grew worse than the day I had arrived. Even friends who are sick are still guests in another's home. As Benjamin Franklin said, "Guests, like fish, begin to smell after three days."

"Sandy's been so nice, amazing really. I just don't want to be a burden, yet I don't know where to go, Alex," I whispered.

"You're right. Sandy's been wonderful, but we need to get you out of here. Come to my place. It's only a studio, but—"

"That's so far. I don't know if I could handle the drive." I winced, fighting back the pain in my neck. "What about a motel? I don't care how much it costs. There's one near my house."

"That'd be good for a while. I could go back and forth between there and your house to check on the cats and get you whatever you need."

"That sounds like the best option."

Alex called the motel and reserved a room on the bottom floor. He packed my belongings, and we thanked Sandy and her two sons for everything.

Though less than five miles to the motel, every light, sound, and movement on the ride there made me want to vomit. I shut my eyes and pictured a tranquil, turquoise ocean.

Things will get better. They have to.

That was what my instincts told me, and I had every reason to trust them.

chapter sixteen

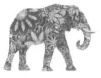

A THING CALLED INSTINCT

MARCH 1991 – SAN DIEGO

I was nineteen, a sophomore in college living in San Diego when I first learned the significance of instincts. My doctor, Dr. Nose Hair, prescribed tetracycline, a general antibiotic, to clear up an infection, instructing me to take one pill three times a day for two weeks.

I filled the prescription and consulted with the pharmacist since I had never taken tetracycline before. As he spoke, I poured a couple of the almond-sized pills into my hand. "These pills are dinosauric, not to mention that the name itself sounds like some sort of flying reptile. How am I supposed to swallow these things?"

"Drink them with lots of water," the pharmacist said, not amused.

I went back to my apartment on campus, poured a full glass of water, and placed a pill on the middle of my tongue, then with my pointer finger, pushed the monstrous pill down to the back of my throat, feeling like a human-sized Pez dispenser. I took a mouthful of water and swallowed hard. The pill went only partway down. I drank at least two glasses full of water before the pill released into my stomach.

Days later, tired from the antibiotics, I skipped classes to rest, continuing to take my gargantuan pills, but each time with less and less water because it grew increasingly more agonizing to swallow. Trying to gulp down a golf ball-sized razor blade dipped in lemon juice would have been more enjoyable. I fell into a weakened state, and my throat started to swell.

I developed the sensation of having a plum pit stuck in the back of my throat. Since my family doctor practiced in L.A., and I had returned to my apartment in San Diego, I went to the campus health center. I needed to finish the antibiotics, but the task appeared unhealthy and daunting.

Dr. Godlike entered the exam room, barely looked at me, then walked over to the window facing a courtyard with students eating lunch, studying, and napping. He looked hairy like a werewolf and smelled like expensive cologne and espresso. "What can I do for you today?"

"Since taking these antibiotics..." I strained to speak. I grasped my throat and continued, "My throat's irritated." I handed him the bottle of pills.

"I see." He looked at the bottle then shook it. "You haven't finished the prescription?"

"There's a week left, but—"

"I suggest you finish the prescription."

"I know...but my throat," I winced. "I didn't hurt before taking these pills. I can't swallow without excruciating pain." A reflex forced me to swallow a pool of saliva. I pointed to my throat, "Maybe...there's something wrong with—"

"There's nothing wrong with you," he snapped. "You need sleep like the rest of the students here. You have to take the remainder of those antibiotics, you hear me?"

"Ah, okay—but could you—at least look at my throat?"

"It looks fine," he said without even glancing up from his clipboard.

"But—"

"I'm the doctor here. I know what I'm talking about." Dr. Godlike grimaced and then left the room.

He didn't even examine me. I've had better medical assistance and advice watching Bugs Bunny reruns. I went home to my apartment, took another prehistoric dosage, and slept for the rest of the day. I became frailer and rarely ate, only drinking water when I forced down the medication.

Something felt wrong, but I went against my own better judgment and listened to that doctor. I had been taught to trust physicians. Still in my teenage years and a rudimentary student of life, who was I to argue?

The next day, I passed out on the carpet next to the coffee table in the living room trying to make my way to the kitchen. Sophie, my fun-loving and kindhearted roommate, who stood four-feet-eleven-inches tall and had the strength and stamina of someone twice her size, found me not long after and brought me to the hospital.

The examining physician, Dr. Hero, looked like a cross between a jockey and a devoted sci-fi fan. He was concerned about me, especially since my throat was swollen and tender to his delicate palpation.

I hunched over on a stool in an examination room that looked more like a medical supply closet. A table of cleaning supplies, tubs of bleach, and clean linens stood in a corner, and the loud buzzing of a machine echoed behind me.

His voice came soft. "Cherie, I realize this will be painful, but I have to scope your throat to see what's going on."

I nodded, hoping the word "scope" referred to mouthwash.

A nurse came in wheeling a tray with a number of shiny instruments on it. None of them looked like anything I wanted to become more intimate with, and there was no minty-fresh mouth rinse in sight.

"It's important you remain still during this procedure, relaxing as much as possible to avoid possible perforation."

Perforate? I never thought a term used around an office supply store would sound so alarming.

The nurse helped the doctor into a pair of latex gloves and handed him the largest, most intrusive looking of all the instruments from the tray.

He leaned toward me. "Okay, open up, really wide. Now, on the count of three, we are going to slip the scope down your throat. One, two, three...."

Thirty minutes later my raw, defiled throat and the rest of me lay upon a stiff metal table. The doctor returned and rested his hand on my shoulder. "Cherie, how you doing?"

Tears formed in my eyes. I forced an artificial grin.

"I know you're in a lot of pain. I spoke with some of my colleagues and none of us have ever seen anything like this before. It seems those antibiotics lodged in your throat, and your stomach acid came up into your esophagus to dissolve them. The acids have caused seven ulcers in your esophagus. We need to admit you into the hospital."

The doctor and nurse helped me into a wheelchair and escorted me through the main portion of the hospital to a large, empty patient room. Two nurses lifted me into a bed, changed me into a gown, and started an IV drip.

Once the IV was in place, the doctor came in.

"We're going to give you some morphine through your IV. It'll give you relief and help you relax."

"How can we get rid of them?" I asked in a nervous whisper.

"There's nothing we can do to treat them. They have to heal on their own. The IV will nourish you since you can't eat anything while they're healing. Also, it's imperative you don't drink anything, not even water. Don't even brush your teeth. Nothing should pass down your throat. We need that area left alone to heal."

A nurse hung up a clear bag next to my IV and fed the two lines together into my arm. With the flick of a plastic switch, the morphine entered my veins and all of my pain vanished. *WEEEEEEEE*, said my brain.

This stuff is fabulous. Why didn't you give me this earlier?

The doctor continued talking, but his words sounded like Charlie Brown's teachers. Wha wha wha wha, wha. Whatever you say, Doc.

I don't care about anything right now. This morphine is almost worth getting ulcers in my esophagus...almost.

For five days of IV bags and morphine, I slithered in and out of sleep until my private drug-induced state was interrupted by an older woman who was placed in the bed across from me.

She got food, drinks, and ice cream. I watched her, salivating, longing for even one drop of water, one taste of food. After not eating or drinking for almost a week, I craved anything.

I watched at mealtimes, my mouth empty and lonely, while she took a bite of the mystery stew, complaining to the nurses about the horrid taste. To me, it looked like a gourmet feast. I would have probably even eaten Fancy Feast cat food at that moment.

Even more than food, I craved water. Parched beyond any sensible comprehension, my lips and throat felt shriveled and dried out. Even the cracks in my lips started to bleed. The dry, soured taste in my mouth felt horrendous, like someone had shoved soiled gym socks in my mouth and put duct tape across my lips. The Gobi desert that posed as my mouth nudged me to drink something, even camel urine if it was available.

Despite the explicit instructions by the doctor not to eat or drink anything, the nurses kept bringing me trays of food and glasses of water. Each time I had to thank them, but remind them, "I'm not supposed to have anything. Please stop bringing me stuff."

Every time this happened the nurse acted surprised and made a notation on my chart. Sometimes they acted proud and brought me a tray with soup, Jell-O, and a glass of water, thinking a liquid diet would be suitable. Each time I turned down the edible items, pissing off my taste buds and stomach.

By the end of my first week in the hospital, the doctor tapered me off the morphine. Welcome to withdrawals.

After ten days, I was drug-free and swallowing almost normally. One final examination concluded the ulcers had cleared, and I was free to go home.

After meeting Dr. Hero and the kind hospital staff who had cared for me, I thought about Dr. Godlike. I wanted to see him and explain what happened to show him the effects of what he had done (or rather, had *not* done), but it was only a fleeting thought. It wasn't like me to seek confrontation. Besides, I had more important things to do, like sleep.

My friends welcomed me with flowers, a feast of pizza, salad, garlic bread, and a large pitcher of ice water. A sign that my roommate Sophie wrote read, "For Cherie."

I felt so much love. "Ah, thank you guys! This is wonderful!"

They gathered around and watched as I drank enough water to fill Lake Superior, but I only ate two bites of pizza and one bite of salad. My stomach felt full immediately. It took weeks before I ate normally again, but right from the moment I arrived home, I couldn't stop drinking water or brushing my teeth. I threw out the Scope mouthwash I had in the medicine cabinet. I couldn't bear to look at it. Just that word "scope" gave me the willies.

chapter seventeen

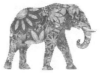

UPROOTED

MAY 2004 – SAN DIEGO

I studied the stained, drab beige motel walls and the floral bedspread underneath me. The phone book and tourist brochures for San Diego sat near a large television mounted to the top of a dresser.

While Alex ran errands, I sat alone with my wandering thoughts, trying to make sense of the day. How long would I endure this suffering?

The room closed in around me. The cheap artwork, lopsided lamps, and generic toiletries laced with the smell of cleaning products and instant coffee. The vast world outside the walls was a universe beyond mine, all far out of my reach.

I thought about the decisions we make and the realities we create as human beings. We wake up, there is a day before us—a canvas of white to compose our unique picturesque life. We strive, overwhelm, idealize, drift, accept, and reject. We may fight back, take back, give back, give in, or give up. We might even save a life, take a life, retreat into mediocrity, or do nothing.

I envisioned the millions of people parading around the planet with active purpose while my life stalled, powerless and inert. I questioned my existence and ability to rise above my helplessness. I wanted to believe I possessed the power to escape.

My pulse throbbed underneath my skin. For three days, I rolled back and forth on the stiff bed, struggling to find comfortable positions. Alex came and went, since he not only tended to me, but juggled a variety of other responsibilities, including work and caring for my cats.

"I want to go home, Alex." I stared at the evergreen-colored carpet, feeling consumed with desperation. He sat on a chair near the window, typing on his laptop.

"You can't. Can you make it to my place?"

My heart stammered thinking of being in a car, my senses to be assaulted by noises, sights, and sounds. The bitter taste of acid leapt into my throat. "What about my boys?" I referred to my cats as "my boys" since I considered them my furry little children.

"Don't worry. I'll take care of them. Let's get you to my place."

Both my cats were male. Actually, one was a hermaphrodite who was both spayed and neutered. The veterinarian said he was one in a million, which was one of the reasons why no one would adopt him. The other reason was because he was black. Apparently, black cats are the least wanted. The thought saddened me.

An all-black double-gender kitty wasn't on the top of the list for adoption. Having a tender spot for unwanted animals, I adopted him, a sleek, barely one-year-old feline I named Ducatti since his purr roared like a finely tuned motorcycle, spelled with two "tt's" to differentiate him from the machine.

My other kitty was an eight-year-old named Mr. Riley. I had rescued him after he was rejected from several homes because he wasn't playful enough. I don't think anyone gave him much of a chance, since he was the sweetest, most adorable creature I'd ever met. He sported a tan, tiger-striped coat and possessed the most lovable disposition. After being with me for a couple of weeks, he played like a kitten. Silly humans.

At the inception of my illness, Ducatti (Duke for short) and I had been together for over five years and Riley and I for almost two. Although I felt concerned about their well-being, Alex loved animals, particularly cats. I needed to focus on getting healthy and finding a way to reunite with my four-legged sons.

The bumpy freeway ride in Alex's Jeep from the motel to his studio apartment knocked me to and fro. My muscles tightened. I stared into the dimness of my eyelids, concentrating on my shallow breaths. Alex carried me upstairs into his four-hundred-square-foot apartment that had one bed, a brown couch, a pine coffee table, and a television nestled on top of the Styrofoam packaging it came in. His simple square kitchen fit only one person. There was a child-sized bathroom. He had no decorations. The room appeared devoid of style, yet a huge step up from the motel room and big enough for what I needed to do—sleep.

Alex placed me on his bed and sat on the couch across from me. My eyes grew droopy, and I succumbed to my first slumber in over a week. Alex stayed close by, working on his laptop from the couch.

A loud noise coming from outside his only window startled me, and I woke.

Alex stood. "Just some kids playing outside. How you doing, CK?"

I relaxed and looked up at him. "Hey."

His kind blue eyes sparkled in the sunlight. I felt myself safe with him, and in that moment I felt no discomfort, only the depth of his affection. I wondered how hard this was for him, aiding me, not knowing what to expect next. He barely knew me, yet he acted like we had been in each other's lives for decades.

As I became more aware of my surroundings, I felt all of my symptoms returning. "I don't think anything has changed."

"You think you'll be all right for an hour or two while I check on the boys and get us something to eat?" Alex asked.

"I think so."

"I'll be back soon. I have my cell. Call if you need me."

"Okay. Thank you. And Alex?"

"Yes?"

"You're wonderful."

Alex kissed me on my lips and left.

I thought about the upcoming tests, the insufferable waiting, and the inevitable results. The path before me looked tiresome.

But the not knowing what was wrong with me was the most deplorable part.

Within one week, I endured MRIs; CAT scans; X-rays; blood, urine, and saliva tests. With every test, I hoped to get closer to understanding my illness.

A couple of days after completing the tests, Alex and I waited in Dr. Friendly's office. Alex typed on his Blackberry, and I focused on breathing while studying several diplomas and accolades that hung on the wall behind the doctor's desk.

"Hello again, Cherie. How are you?" Dr. Friendly, the neurologist, shook my hand. My heart started pounding when I saw him holding my chart with my test results.

"What did you find, doctor?"

He leaned against his desk. "As I suspected, everything came back normal."

"How could that be?" Alex asked.

"Normal?" I motioned to my unstable, shaking, and contorted body with my hands. "This is not normal."

"Your symptoms are not normal, but I'm not surprised by the results." The doctor flipped through the chart. "These tests rule out several possible candidates for your ailments. This was a wide spectrum of tests, but there are many others we can do. Also, I think it would be good for you to see a physical medicine specialist who handles cases like yours with inconclusive test results and an array of clear clinical symptoms."

Alex rubbed his temples. "What about the mold in her house, and the malaria she had?"

"Her malaria test was negative, but that doesn't mean it's gone. Although I think she needs to move, I don't think the mold is her main problem, but rather, a contributing factor to a larger issue."

I sighed. "So you have no idea what's wrong with me?"

"Not at this point. I'll write you a recommendation for the other specialist and a script for more tests. We'll have to keep looking."

Over the next few weeks, while waiting for more tests results and approval from my insurance, what I truly waited for was my life to be given back to me.

I tucked the blankets under my chin and studied Alex sitting on the couch typing on his laptop. He had dark circles beneath his eyes and he looked thin. "Alex, you have a minute?"

"Sure." He set his laptop on the coffee table and sat next to me. "What do you need?"

"I've been living on your couch for a few weeks. I was at Sandy's and the motel for almost a week before that. I thought I would know what was happening to me by now."

"I know, CK, it's frustrating, but we have to keep—"

"I appreciate everything you're doing. You've been wonderful, I can't thank you enough, but I can't keep doing this. My rent's due for June and my cats have been alone for almost a month. I need to think about moving out and getting an apartment. I want to be with my boys, have my clothes and stuff."

"It is ridiculous to pay rent for a place you're not even using, and an unhealthy one at that."

"You think the landlord will let me out of the lease?"

"Don't worry. I'll take care of it."

I was certain of my love for Alex, so devoted, so caring. What I wanted most was to heal so I could give him the affection and care he deserved.

Alex called my roommate from college, Sophie, the one that helped me when I had ulcers in my esophagus, and one of the first and best friends I had made when I moved to San Diego. Now married, she and her husband, Jason, were a big part of my life.

Sophie helped me find an apartment that was affordable, close to work, clean, and mold-free. The apartment was also tucked away from any main streets, so it would be quiet and safe for me and my cats, far away from the coyote-infested canyons in northern San Diego.

Alex, Sophie, and Jason packed, moved, and unpacked everything I owned. By the middle of June, all my "Bs"—my being, my boys, and my belongings—were moved out of Alex's studio and my disease-ridden, rundown house into my new apartment.

After the move, Alex helped me throw away several items that had mold on them. Dr. Friendly recommended washing anything porous in hot water to eliminate all traces of mold. In my hallway next to my half-sized washer and dryer, Alex piled every item of clothing, towel, and bedding I owned. I spent the first month in my new apartment harnessing a little energy each day to do a small amount of laundry.

Now, ten miles south of my previous place in my new two-bedroom apartment on the bottom floor of a well-manicured complex, I became part of the living—relieved to once again have a home. My cats cuddled near me, purring and keeping me grounded emotionally, but my symptoms remained unchanged.

chapter eighteen

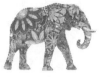

HEARTBROKEN

JUNE 2004 – SAN DIEGO

I sat in my kitchen, dialing the phone. "I'm calling to make an appointment to see a physiatrist. My neurologist referred me."

"Hold on a moment," a robust female voice said. I loved being put on hold—my newest hobby. "Okay. What do you need to be seen for?"

"I've been sick for six weeks. I'm hoping the physiatrist will—"

"What's your diagnosis?"

"I don't have one."

"We need a diagnosis to schedule you. What should I put?"

"The reason I'm coming to your office is to get a diagnosis."

"I can't schedule you without one."

My heart beat faster. "Isn't a physiatrist a pain specialist?"

"That's correct."

I took a breath. "I'm in pain every day and all night. So please, put whatever you need to so I can see her."

"Fine. Her first opening's next Friday at 3 p.m. We'll see you then." Click.

The next morning, I woke from a haunting nightmare of being back in Zambia, sick and alone in the wilderness, dying. No one was around to help me. My legs had been amputated. I had no way to find help. I smelled charcoal in the air and felt the darkness of death suffocating my breath as my blood drained through the holes where my legs used to be.

I gasped and sat up in bed, clutching my knees to my chest. The sensations from my nightmare were still so vivid it took me a few

137

moments to realize where I was. I got up and splashed cold water on my face. I was in my new apartment in San Diego with my two beautiful cats. Ducatti was sleeping at the foot of my bed, but I couldn't find Riley. I searched the whole apartment, and waited all day, my heart racing, watching the cat door for his return. He didn't come home.

After dinner, I called Alex. "Riley's missing."

"Missing?"

"He was scratching at the cat door early this morning. He was relentless, so I opened it and he ran straight out. He never strays far past the patio."

"He's not back yet? It's almost 6 p.m." Alex sounded worried.

"I've called him and looked around the apartment, but I can't walk far. Can you look for him?"

"I'll be right there."

Alex arrived with a flashlight and a plastic toy with a tiny metal bell inside. He scoured the apartment complex for Riley until late into the night, but still no sign of him.

Riley was a gentle, timid feline. His previous pet parent had had him declawed, so he could not defend himself. I needed to find him.

Days later, Riley had still not returned. I made flyers, which Alex posted around the neighborhood, and he continued to look for Riley every chance he could. I stayed home, awaiting his return. He was still missing on the day of my appointment.

I waited in what looked more like a lounge than a doctor's office. Soothing classical musical played, abstract oil paintings decorated the walls, and a bamboo plant in a green ceramic pot sat in the center of a table next to my chair. My friend Bruce had driven me to my appointment and sat next to me. He was a rugged-looking man with a tall, athletic frame, sporting a navy flannel shirt, full beard and mustache. As he flipped through a cycling magazine, I recalled how we had met working at a software company a few years before. At lunch we'd gone for walks, rode bikes, and enjoyed time in nature. He was much like Alex—from the East Coast, a highly intellectual, reclusive engineer who befriended few people. But we bonded instantly, one of those unexplainable connections, like someone you felt you'd known all your life.

The first time Alex met Bruce and his wife, Rebecca, was for lunch at their house in the secluded area of Ramona. They lived off a dirt road. Their house had two stories and a wrap-around balcony overlooking miles of open land sprinkled with farms and houses.

During lunch, our conversation turned into a discussion on the goodness of people. Alex said, "Cherie's too kind and optimistic about people. She thinks everyone has good intentions and that they're inherently moral and nice."

"What's wrong with that?" I said.

Rebecca smiled, nodding. Rebecca was an artist, an athletic and natural woman who had a smile that lit up any room.

Bruce smirked at Rebecca and me. "You're both so naive." His New York accent sounded faint.

"Seventy-five percent of the people in the world are assholes," Alex said, as if stating a well-researched statistic.

Bruce slicked back his mustache and beard with his fingers. "That number's way too low. It's more like ninety-five percent."

Alex and Bruce laughed in unison. They too were instant friends.

I was brought back into the moment in the waiting room by the familiar sensation that someone was looking at me. It was Bruce. The cycling magazine folded in his hand. His eyebrows furrowed.

I turned in my chair toward him. "What is it?"

"I was just thinking about our bike rides together. I miss them."

I sighed.

"Don't worry, Cherie. We'll do 'em again someday."

"Yeah. And hey, you still owe me another ride on your tractor!"

"Of course. You can even drive it." He flashed me a broad and handsome smile.

I smiled back, feeling honored. I knew what a big deal that was for him. Bruce loved his tractor as much as I loved my cats. And even though we never said it, I knew Bruce and I cared deeply for each other. And I knew we would always be friends.

"Thanks for driving me here."

"Don't mention it. I'm selfish. I want you back cycling again."

My thoughts drifted to one of our cycling adventures. We had snuck out of work for an extended lunch hour. Bruce led us down a hilly dirt trail near our office. He maneuvered a tight turn and flew fast down a long, rocky hill. I strained to keep up with him. Although adept on a bike, I wasn't the daredevil type. I gripped the handles, my hands poised over the brakes. Sweat trickled down my back.

Bruce took another tight turn. I followed, but felt like I was going too fast. I pressed hard on the brakes. I skidded, my bike slipped out to the side, and I flew off and slid on the coarse path. "Ah!" I screamed.

Bruce heard my crash, turned his bike around, and rode back to me. He got off his bike, knelt down, and extended his hand. "You alright?"

"Yeah, I think so. I'm just not as fast as you." I grabbed his hand and he pulled me up.

"Well, what you lack in speed, you make up for in other ways."

"I'll take that as a compliment."

"It is. You know I only have a few friends. And you're one."

I smiled while I brushed off dirt from my legs.

"I'll slow down a bit. Okay?"

"Thanks, Bruce. That'd be great."

An unfamiliar voice calling out my name brought me back into the moment in the waiting lounge. Minutes later I was escorted into a private exam room, and shortly after the physiatrist entered the room and closed the door. Her long dark hair and deep brown eyes contrasted with her white physician's coat. "I'm Dr. Polite."

"Nice to meet you, doctor." I smelled vanilla-scented lotion as we shook hands.

"Cherie, I've reviewed all of the reports and test results from your primary doctor and neurologist. I'd like to find out more of your medical history and conduct an examination. Why are you holding your neck like that?"

I fidgeted. "Pain, but also my neck can't support my head."

"Can you put your hands down for a minute while I examine you?"

"I'll try. But it would be best if I lie down."

"Why don't you stand up, will that be any easier?"

"I have trouble standing. I get stabbing left-sided headaches, and I get dizzy and out of breath." My hands shook.

"How'd you get here today?"

"My friend Bruce took the afternoon off work to drive me."

Dr. Polite smiled. "He's a great friend."

"Indeed. I don't know what I'd do without my friends. I rely on them for everything."

"You don't have any family close by?"

"No. But my boyfriend, he's been so devoted."

"I'm glad you have someone to help you." Dr. Polite smiled again then placed cold, soft hands on my neck. "Try and hold still."

Later that night, I could not stop shaking. I felt hungry and tired, but was looking forward to seeing Alex, who was bringing dinner.

"It's open, honey," I said from my usual fetal position on the couch. I had unlocked it the last time I had to get up to use the bathroom. I limited the frequency of trips off the couch or out of bed. If I did too much, I had trouble breathing. My muscles would shake and cramp. Sometimes I collapsed.

Alex sat next to me on the floor and kissed me on the cheek. "How you feeling?"

"The same."

"How about Riley?"

"He's not back. I'm so worried about him."

"We'll find him." Alex paused, as if saying a silent prayer for my lost cat. "How did it go at the physiatrist's office today?"

"Let's eat first. I don't want the food to get cold."

"Don't worry about the food. What did the doctor say?"

"She said I've been through a considerable amount of trauma for someone my age, which I already knew, though hearing it from a doctor was strangely validating."

"Did she have any idea what's wrong with you?"

I took in a long breath. "She said I have fibromyalgia. It's primarily muscular pain and tightness."

"It doesn't sound like a solid diagnosis."

"She sounded more like she was guessing than knowing."

"Are there any tests to find out whether you have it or not?"

"They look for tender spots on the body. Apparently I have ten out of thirteen. She also mentioned chronic fatigue syndrome."

"You are exhausted."

"She said these are symptoms, not diseases. She believes I have both, but that I have more of a systemic problem that tests aren't showing."

"What'd she recommend?"

"A rheumatologist." I held back my tears. "Can we eat now? I don't want to talk about it anymore tonight."

He put his arm around my shoulders. "We're going to figure this out. You have a follow-up appointment with the cardiologist tomorrow to do a stress test and heart ultrasound. Maybe that will show something."

I appreciated Alex's optimism, since he was usually such a pessimist. I wondered if he honestly believed I could find answers and heal.

"You're so good to me." I smiled but wanted to cry, not only for my suffering, but for Alex and all he endured.

"You're a wonderful person, Cherie. You deserve to be healthy, and you deserve my help."

I questioned whether my torment was karma teaching me some sort of lesson: that I deserved to suffer.

He helped me sit up, and I picked at my food, eating only because I had to. I had already lost too much weight, but I lacked the energy or motivation to chew.

A couple of days later, as I forced down breakfast, the phone rang.

"Ms. Kephart?" said a woman, with a raspy voice I did not recognize. "This is Veronica, Dr. Calm's nurse from the Cardiology Center. He reviewed your test results and asked me to call you right away."

Nervous, I sat up on the couch. "What is it?"

"I called in a prescription for you. You need to pick it up and start taking it right away. Your test results show several episodes of supraventricular tachycardia, or SVT."

"SVT?"

"Your heart rate is dramatically sped up by an abnormal electrical impulse starting in the atria. It's beating so fast that the heart muscle can't relax between contractions. When these chambers don't relax, they can't fill with enough blood to provide for the body's needs. Because of the ineffective contractions, the brain doesn't receive enough blood and oxygen. You're often lightheaded and dizzy, right?"

"All the time."

"Those are symptoms related to SVT. It can make you tired, and you can pass out, which is why you need medication. It may be an indication of Wolff-Parkinson-White, a syndrome caused by abnormal accessory pathways in the heart. WPW can lead to sudden cardiac death if not treated, but we're not sure that's what you have. We need to get you on this medication to start."

"What about my neurological symptoms, and my stabbing headaches, and all my other symptoms, are they from SVT or WPW?"

"It's doubtful. These heart conditions are more common than people realize, except most people don't have the magnitude and frequency of episodes that you're experiencing. You go into SVT too easily and frequently, which is dangerous, especially with all of your other symptoms. Dr. Calm wants you to be extra careful not to exert yourself and take this new prescription beta blocker. Can you get to the pharmacy today?"

"Yeah, I'll get someone to take me."

"Dr. Calm also wants you to start wearing a heart-rate monitor. I'll have someone call you to set that up."

Hours later, I swayed back and forth in my chair, waiting for the prescription to reach my heart and decrease the speed of my pulse. My mother would be arriving soon from L.A. to take care of me for the weekend; grocery shopping, laundry, cleaning, and making meals. This would be her first visit since I had become ill. How would I tell her I had a heart arrhythmia? I didn't want to cause her any anxiety.

Once she arrived, she sat on the couch and hugged me. I smelled the fragrance of roses on her neck. I leaned against the cushions and studied her fuchsia lipstick, pink blouse, and gold watch wrapped around her pale, petite wrist. She had inherited her parents' brown eyes and hair, and clear, smooth skin, looking much younger than her biological age.

She also hadn't met Alex yet. This was not the way I wanted them to meet.

"Thanks for coming, Mom."

"Of course. I'm worried about you."

"Try not to. I've got wonderful friends. And Alex has been great. He's an amazing man."

"I'm sure he is. I want to thank him." She looked pensive and sad. "I wish you lived closer, I could help more, but with work, and taking care of my dad, I'm so busy."

My grandfather had recently turned ninety. He was in great physical health and still lived alone, but needed my mother's help for lots of things. I was close with him and we spoke on the phone a few times every week, as I did with my mother. They were wonderful about checking up on me, as was my Uncle Jim, and my great Uncles Blaise, Buddy, and Roger. I loved living in San Diego, but I missed my family.

We talked for more than an hour about my health and all of the latest developments, particularly my heart.

"Did the nurse say what caused it?" Her voice sounded loud in my ear.

"No, they aren't sure." I wiped my face with a tissue. "I may have an accessory pathway in my heart. They want me to see an electro-cardiologist."

The doorbell rang.

"You expecting anyone?" my mom asked.

"No."

She walked across the living room, looked through the peep hole, and opened the door. Two young boys wearing soccer uniforms, about seven or eight years old, stood on my welcome mat.

I recognized them. They lived a few apartments down. I often saw them playing soccer. I stood and wobbled toward the door.

"Hi. Can I help you?" One of them had a crumpled piece of paper in his hand. He held it up, straightening it out so I could see. My flyer.

My hopes skyrocketed. "That's my cat. Have you seen him?"

The other child said, "Yes, we just saw him."

My heart skipped. "Where?"

"We found him over there." The first kid pointed toward the front of the apartment complex.

I gasped. "What do you mean you found him?"

The first kid said, "On the grass near the entrance. We found half of him."

"Half?" I shrieked. "Are you sure it's him?" I motioned to the photo of Riley on the paper.

Both kids nodded. "We can show you."

I followed the boys, my feet pressing in the grass behind theirs. I wanted to stop after every few steps, but my surging adrenaline helped me press on. My pulse grew faster, stabbing sensations with each beat.

"Please, let it be a mistake," I said under my breath. "Please, not my Riley."

Closer and closer we walked to a spacious grassy area underneath a tall and expansive white birch tree. From a distance, I saw an unidentifiable lump in a shady part of the lawn. I held my breath.

I paused, and leaned forward. In the blades of grass, I saw the head and torso of a cat, mangled by the jaws and claws of a predator, the lower half of his body missing.

I looked closer. The fur was tan with stripes. No doubt, it was him. "Oh God, no!" I shouted, shaking. "Not my baby!"

The children stood and stared as I fell to my knees and gripped handfuls of grass in my fists and yelled, "Not Riley."

Minutes later, I stumbled back to my apartment.

My mom rushed to my side. "What's wrong?"

"I have to call Alex." I dialed. He answered, and I screamed into the phone, "Riley's dead!"

I dropped the phone and paced back and forth, hysterical with grief. The pace of my heart increased. I felt dizzy and my chest tightened. I hyperventilated.

"Cherie, you need to relax. This isn't good for your heart."

"Relax? He's dead, Mom, Riley's dead!" I shouted. "He was so kind, so pure. He didn't deserve what he got."

My mom's voice rose. "You need to calm down."

"I can't," I barked back at her.

"I know you're upset, but it's going to be okay."

"Okay?" I panted, throwing my arms around in a chaotic motion. "It's not okay. I opened the door. I let him out. He's dead because of me."

I felt like I was going to pass out. My mother helped me to the couch and held me close, stroking my hair like she did when I was a child. I cried in her arms. "I'm sorry, Mom."

"It's okay." She gently rocked me.

My heart felt like it ruptured with each beat. "I love you, Mom. Thank you for being here with me. It means so much."

About thirty minutes later, Alex knocked on the door. My mom answered.

"I'm Alex." He extended his hand to her. She nudged it away and hugged him instead.

chapter nineteen

PAINFULLY SANE

OCTOBER 2004 – SAN DIEGO

Alex opened the front door of my apartment with the spare key I had given him. "You ready?"

I closed my journal and placed it on my desk. "I'll be right there."

Alex and I met in the hallway. He kissed me gently on the lips.

On the car ride, I felt an urge to head home. My primary doctor, Dr. Kind, whom I had been seeing long before this crazy illness, had moved to North Carolina. I trusted her, and she understood me. She used to call me a vibrant woman, but she had also witnessed how this latest illness had struck me down. Dr. Kind was always by my side, assisting to help me find a diagnosis, a cure, and easement for my suffering. She gave me hope, and always supported my efforts to heal. "I still can't believe Dr. Kind is gone. She was such a great doctor."

Alex stayed quiet, his expression one of concern. He knew how devastated I had been the day Dr. Kind told me she was leaving.

"My new doctor was mildly sympathetic at first, but since all the tests keep coming back negative, she's giving me looks like I'm wasting her time and there's nothing wrong with me."

Alex rested his hand on mine. "You're not wasting her time. If anything, she's wasting yours by not continuing to look for ways to help you."

An hour later I was lying on the examination table, waiting for Dr. Loveless. The walls were painted pale blue and filled with posters depicting human anatomy. I studied the poster with the heart, picturing mine pulsing frantically.

A few minutes later, Dr. Loveless entered the room. She was a petite but muscular woman. I had the feeling she could arm wrestle Mike Tyson, if need be.

"Cherie, the latest tests came back normal," she said without much expression. "You're slightly anemic, but you've lost so much weight, which may be a factor."

One hand supported my neck, the other gripped Alex's hand. "What do you think we should try next?"

She sighed and shook her head. "I don't know what other tests to run at this point. You may just have fibromyalgia and chronic fatigue syndrome."

Alex spoke on my behalf. He was used to it now. "She still hasn't been able to see the rheumatologist to confirm those diagnoses."

"Remind me again, why?" Dr. Loveless asked.

Alex explained. "Even with Dr. Kind's referral, her HMO said she's already been diagnosed with fibromyalgia by the physiatrist and Dr. Kind. Because of this, they keep denying her requests, stating she doesn't need to see a specialist."

"I'm appealing it now," I said.

"It's ridiculous," Alex added. "If she has this illness, shouldn't she be approved to see a specialist to confirm the diagnosis and help treat her? What if the physiatrist is right and this is only a symptom, like the fatigue, and perhaps even the SVT, and there's something worse wrong? I can't believe these insurance companies."

"Maybe the insurance company has a point," Dr. Loveless chimed in. "Perhaps it's time we considered this is all you have."

"Dr. Kind, the cardiologist, the neurologist, and the physiatrist all said they believe she has a more systemic problem, they just aren't certain what it is. Her list of symptoms keeps growing: neuropathy, numbness, stomach pain, chest tightening, foot cramps, vertigo."

I pointed to my chest. "I haven't been able to wear a bra in six months; it's too painful. And lately, if I lie on my back, my head feels like it's being sucked through the floor with the extreme G force of a fighter plane."

"She hasn't worked since April," Alex continued. "She can't drive. Her friends and I take care of her. Her mom drives down on weekends. All Cherie can do is lie around in pain waiting for someone to help her."

"What happened with the beta blockers the cardiologist prescribed?" Dr. Loveless asked.

I cleared my throat. "My symptoms got worse, then I tried a calcium blocker, which was unbearable."

"The cardiologist had her stop taking both of those," Alex added. "He said it's common for younger people not to tolerate those types of drugs."

Dr. Loveless looked distracted, glanced at her watch, then asked, "What are they doing for your heart?"

"I'm waiting to see a specialist to go over my heart-rate recordings. I've been wearing the device for a couple of months now."

Dr. Loveless looked down on me. "All I'm saying is that perhaps we should consider trying you on some anti-depressants. You seem stable enough to me." She stepped back, then scribbled on her prescription pad.

You call this stable? I wish everyone would stop saying that.

I took a shallow breath and sat up. "Dr. Loveless, I was depressed once years ago, and I've never felt that way since, not even now with all this pain."

Alex squeezed my hand. "If anything, she's depressed because she's sick."

"I don't want medications to mask my symptoms. I want to get to the root of the problem, not live a dulled existence while watching my physical symptoms get worse. My body's trying to tell me something. Dr. Kind agreed with me on this."

She placed the prescription pad in her coat pocket and folded her arms. "You have to consider that this might be all in your head."

Cherie Kephart

My face and neck felt hot. "You think I'm crazy? That I'm making this up?"

"Sometimes our minds can be so formidable they can cause physical pain."

I tried to remain calm as I spoke, but my heart beat faster and faster. "How would my mind cause my heart to go into SVT? When I get muscle cramps, my big toe springs outward, practically separating itself from my foot. I've started getting red, splotchy rashes on my chest, and my neck has the strength and elasticity of Jell-O lined with serrated knives. Each time I turn or move in a way my body doesn't like, I get cut internally. How could these symptoms be solely in my mind?"

Dr. Loveless headed toward the door. "I can't help you if you're not willing to try what I recommend."

"That's all I've been doing for the past six months. Prescriptions, acupuncture, herbs, supplements, osteopathic and chiropractic treatments, meditation CDs, relaxation techniques, and physical therapy. Everything has either not helped or made me worse. Everyone's guessing. I want to find out what's causing these symptoms so I can treat the problem, not cover it up and hide behind chemicals. If I cover up my symptoms, I may never heal. I want to be healthy again."

Dr. Loveless shrugged.

"Trust me, Dr. Loveless, I am painfully sane."

She started out the door. With Alex's help I stood. "Should I come back in two weeks?"

"Why don't we start spreading out the appointments to a month," she said, and then left.

I watched her walk down the hall, realizing I'd never see her again.

150

chapter twenty

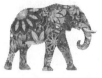

DESPERATE TIMES

NOVEMBER 2004 – LOS ANGELES

I was beyond desperate, which is how Vladimir came into my life.

"I can't believe it's been almost seven months I've been sick," I said to Alex. "I don't know what I'd do without you."

He smiled. His hands gripped the steering wheel of his Jeep, his focus on the road. Our affection for each other continued to expand. I had unconditional support and friendship from Alex. I am not certain what he saw in me, and I dared not think about what would happen if he were not there. I believed in many ways I was alive because of him.

"I love you, Alex."

"And I love you, CK."

We had recently started saying I love you to one another. It felt right. Even though our romantic relationship was on hold because of my health, our bond and mutual respect grew. Alex wanted to focus on my health, and then think about our relationship once I was better. I agreed and looked forward to the day when I was healed and we could resume what we had started.

"Do you think Vladimir's going to help me?"

"I'm skeptical." Alex was a conventional kind of guy who looked for concrete evidence. He wasn't much on intuition or serendipity, two of my favorite words.

"My friend Sally said he helped her."

"Your Peace Corps buddy?"

"Yes. We always have a good laugh about how our experiences were so different. I was in one of the most rural, disease-ridden places on the earth, digging wells and latrines and trying to prevent people, including myself, from dying, while she taught sports and recreation to children on a little island in the Caribbean."

I took a couple of breaths. "Her biggest worry as a Peace Corps volunteer was skin cancer because she tanned herself on white sandy beaches where she sipped rum punch and ate freshly caught lobster."

"Boy, you got screwed on your assignment."

I giggled.

"Would you do it all again, knowing what you know now?"

I recalled Fewdays and the villagers of Mulundu. "I want to say yes, but if I'm honest, I doubt it. I hate being this sick. I feel cheated, and I wonder how my life would be if I had taken another path. Maybe that's what's wrong with me. Some foreign disease the medical community doesn't have a name for."

"You just saw that infectious disease specialist, Dr. Bloodsucker. All those elaborate tests came back negative."

I sighed. "Yeah, but Dr. Bloodsucker said there are many diseases that are difficult to detect through lab tests, and the malaria's still with me. He said it will never go away. It's suppressing my immune system. Maybe that could cause all of this?"

"I don't know. Tell me again what this guy Vladimir does."

I stared out the window watching cars pass us. "All I know is that he's an energetic healer, moved here from Russia where he was supposedly a renowned physicist."

"And now he lives in Hollywood, works out of his apartment, and charges $150 an hour. Cash only."

"I know it sounds odd, but Sally has her master's in public health from UCLA and teaches health and nutrition at a public high school. This healer can't be too far off the deep end."

Vladimir's worn-down apartment was tucked away between several other old buildings in North Hollywood. The air around his neighborhood felt thicker, as if the smog of L.A. liked to settle there.

Alex and I arrived, greeted by Vladimir's wife, who spoke no English. She pointed to the tattered tweed couch to the left of the front door and motioned for us to sit, then went to the kitchen, sat on a tall breakfast stool, ate dry cereal from a box, and watched soap operas from a small black-and-white television mounted on the wall.

The room felt stuffy and smelled like sauerkraut. The curtains were drawn, and the dim light in the room illuminated the peeling green wallpaper. We waited almost an hour before Vladimir appeared.

Well into his sixties, Vladimir was a short, stubby man with more silver hair than black. He wore indigo scrubs, white tennis shoes, and a gold chain around his neck. His robust Russian accent dwarfed his English. He walked his last patient to the front door, then turned around and introduced himself to me. He motioned for us to follow him, and yelled something in Russian to his wife.

"Come, come," he said, escorting us into a cramped, cluttered office with hundreds of books and trinkets that hadn't been dusted in decades, if ever. The door creaked as he closed it.

"Sit, sit," he said as he sat. There were only two chairs in the room. I sat in the second chair; Alex stood.

"Oh-kay. Tell me what is wrong with you." Vladimir folded his hands across his chest.

I gave Alex a wan smile, knowing how much I relied on him. By now he was as familiar with recounting my medical history as I was, and without having to say a word in request, he began telling it to Vladimir. He spoke for almost half the hour, while Vladimir listened and took notes.

Suddenly, Vladimir stood and pointed to me. "Enough. Come. Come, here."

I stood next to him, holding my head with my hands. He examined me, touching me all over, as if his hands acquired data, then he pointed to the clock on the wall. My hour was up.

"Oh-kay. Come back next week, da? I will help you, you will see. I know what to do."

"Next week?" I sighed, discouraged. I then said more than I had the entire visit. "I live in San Diego. It's difficult to get here. Do you have any other times sooner? I want to get started."

"Wait. You wait," he told us as he stepped out. After two minutes of yelling in Russian to his wife, he re-entered the room.

"Come back tomorrow. Four and five. Two hours tomorrow. Da?"

I nodded.

Alex didn't look impressed, and I didn't blame him, but he was willing to support my trying different things since he had witnessed many medical doctors shaking their heads and giving up.

When we arrived the next day, Vladimir took us back to the same dust-filled room. There were still only two chairs, but this time I wasn't sitting.

"Cherie, stand front of me," Vladimir said. He wasn't much for salutations or small talk. At $150 an hour, neither was I.

Alex sat and observed. Vladimir, wearing the identical outfit from the day before, stood facing me and placed his hands on my shoulders.

"Relax. All will be fine. We will first work here." He pointed toward my chest with both of his hands.

Since my illness had begun, my breasts and all of the muscles surrounding my chest, rib cage, and upper back and neck had felt knotted and constricted. I couldn't wear a bra or anything snug around my chest because it restricted my breathing. Luckily, my breasts are not too big. Yes, there are pluses to having a smaller chest: I could run, swim, cycle, and play sports without any problems—nothing an enterprising sports bra couldn't handle—and lastly, I knew a guy liked me for me, not for my breasts.

"We must help here, your breathing. This tight, da?" he signaled to my breasts.

"Yes."

"Please. Take off your shirt."

I looked over at Alex. He raised his right eyebrow. I wasn't sure why I needed to have my shirt off, but I complied, since I had a thin tank top on underneath.

154

Vladimir raised his hands, warmed them together, and conducted a series of hand motions around and over my breasts, particularly my left breast, since the left side of my body had the majority of pain and tenseness.

He circled his hand on my left breast, cupped it and moved his fingers in a sweeping motion, then brought his hand away from me and shook his wrist and fingers as if he were throwing away cobwebs from my chest. Sometimes he touched my breasts. Sometimes just the air around them. I shook and fought back tears the entire time. Standing for five minutes unsupported felt like a monumental task, let alone for two hours.

"Oh-kay, we are done," Vladimir announced and left the room.

Alex grabbed my shirt off the floor and handed it to me. I placed it over my head. I couldn't believe what I was feeling. My chest didn't ache, it wasn't tight, and I could breathe deeply.

I paid Vladimir the $300 and scheduled another double appointment for the following week.

As we left the building, I shook with discomfort from my lethargy but I also trembled from elation. This was the first time in six months anyone or anything had alleviated any of my symptoms. Although my neck, shoulders, back, legs, and arms still ached, my breasts and rib cage felt free.

On the return trip to San Diego, Alex drove while I reclined in the passenger's seat with my eyes closed, reflecting on what had occurred. Vladimir did not explain what he did. He used no instruments, no healing herbs or remedies, only the energy from his hands, and the evidence of his energetic healing was in the results. I had entered his office with fibro-cystic breasts, and chest muscles hard as granite. After three sessions, my breasts felt supple and soft and my chest freed from a prison of rigidity.

The next week, I returned for another series of appointments where Vladimir repeated most of what he had done the week before; however, this time he had me lie flat on a table while he orchestrated a symphony of air particles over me, sweeping, waving, and moving his hands. My mother came with me and sat in the corner on a plastic chair watching this stranger help her youngest daughter heal. At the beginning of the appointment, she smiled and told me, "You're going to be fine, Cherie. I love you."

Tears formed in my eyes. "I love you too, Mom."

Two hours passed, and I thanked him for his time and scheduled more appointments for the following week. I hadn't noticed any improvements in my condition, but my chest still felt good, so I decided to keep seeing him, to find out what else he could do to help me.

The next week Alex came and Vladimir repeated most of the movements from the previous sessions. Before we left, he told me he wanted to work on my heart next week, which delighted me because I felt scared about having a rapid heart rate.

"You bring something with you next time," he said.

"Certainly. What?"

"Eggs."

"Did you say eggs?"

"Da. They must be chicken eggs."

A little strange, but I decided not to ask. "I can do that."

"They must be fresh."

"I can pick some up at the store—"

"No, no. Must be fresh. Ah, how do you say?" Vladimir left the room, shouted something in Russian, then came back. "Ah, not fresh, fer-tile. Not one, six chicken eggs. Fertile. Not kind at store. Now go."

He ushered me out the door and escorted his next patient in.

Alex and I walked to his Jeep. "What do you think he needs fertile chicken eggs for?" I asked.

"How would I know?"

"I don't care. He's the only one to help me so far. I have to get them and see where this goes. You with me?"

"It's up to you, Cherie."

"You don't believe in anything he's done, do you?"

"I can't dispute what you've told me. Your breathing rate and your chest symptoms have decreased. He's done more than all the other people you've seen combined, I'll give him that, but he hasn't helped you since that first week. Since then, nothing's improved."

"Maybe it takes time. And eggs."

Locating fertile chicken eggs in L.A. was not easy. I searched the Internet and called every grocery store, conventional and otherwise, but no one sold, carried, or knew of anyone that sold fertile chicken eggs.

After five days of searching, I called Vladimir to tell him my dilemma. Trying to discern his speech in person was difficult, but he was impossible to understand over the telephone. He kept repeating, "Bring the eggs, da? And bring them the same day you buy them."

I attempted to locate a farm in the city of Los Angeles, but the contradiction in that sentence alone was enough to make me and everyone I called laugh.

On the sixth day, I found a rural family business more than an hour drive east of Hollywood that sold fertile chicken eggs.

The man on the phone asked me, "What do you want them for? Are you going to raise chickens?"

I didn't want to risk messing up. I needed the eggs, and needed to sound credible. "I'm a school teacher. As a class project we are going to put them in an incubator and watch them develop and hatch into little chicks."

"How many do you want? They come in cases of twenty-four."

"I only need six."

"We only sell them in cases."

"How about I pay for the full case, and you can donate the rest to the next customer? What time do you open?"

Alex and I drove two hours from San Diego the night before, then another two hours from my mother's place to the store, battling the early morning rush-hour traffic. The store was in an out-of-the-way, rural town. An eerie feeling swept over me. The place looked part ghost town, part sci-fi thriller.

I entered what looked like an old general store. A man in a tan cowboy hat with a large mustache stood behind the counter writing something.

I cleared my throat. "Hi. I'm here for the fertile chicken eggs. I called yesterday."

"Oh yeah, I remember you. What grade are they in?" The man packaged the eggs and rang up my purchase.

"Grade?" I couldn't focus on anything but the chicken eggs.

"Your students?"

"Oh, my students. Yes, them. Ah, first."

"That's pretty young to be learning about this stuff."

"I believe in starting them early. We done here?" I reached for the eggs.

The man handed them to me and gave me an odd look.

With one hand holding my neck, and the other the eggs, I left the store. Alex opened the Jeep door and helped me and my six new acquaintances inside.

We arrived at Vladimir's apartment. Alex carried the eggs because I was shaking and in no position to handle them. The last thing we needed was to drop them.

Vladimir approached us with steam. "You bring eggs, da?"

"Da." I pointed at the tray in Alex's hands. I guess Vladimir was rubbing off on me.

"Good, good. Come, bring them."

By this time, we knew our positions in the room, but we didn't know what to expect. Alex sat, and I stood waiting.

One by one, Vladimir took each chicken egg, in the most delicate of fashions, and held it next to my heart. In silence, he waved it around and pushed it against my chest. He continued the same motions with all six eggs. The entire process took almost the whole hour. "Oh-kay, done," he announced.

"What did the eggs do?" I asked, bursting with curiosity.

"Rhythm of eggs reset pace of your heart to when you were baby."

"But, my heart's still racing, I don't feel any different."

"This takes time. Also, you're not done."

Not done? What else did I have to do, find the parents to each of the eggs and reunite the chicken families?

"Take eggs home. You must destroy them, but they cannot crack or break."

"How are we supposed to destroy them if we can't break them?" Alex asked.

"Burn them," he answered, nonchalantly.

"Do you mean boil them?" I asked.

"No, burn them. Your heart rate will take their rhythms, but if they break, this won't work."

Alex and I didn't know what to say. We paid Vladimir. The money spent totaled well over $1,000, not including the expense of the eggs or gasoline. I had used all the money in my savings to pay for these and other treatments that my insurance wouldn't cover.

We drove to my mother's house in West L.A. Once we arrived, we carried the eggs into her backyard and set them on the concrete slab between the house and the detached garage. Fortunately, my mother was at work. I didn't want to explain what we were about to do.

We paused. Looked at each other. Looked at the eggs. Looked at each other again, then back at the eggs. "How are we going to do this?" I finally asked Alex.

"Don't look at me. This is your show."

I hobbled around to the side of the house and found a small old metal trash can. Alex brought it to the concrete area and lined the bottom of it with newspaper, twigs, and a couple of pieces of scrap wood from my mom's basement. One by one, we cradled the eggs in the newspaper then found matches in the house.

Alex, Mr. Safety, uncoiled the garden hose and got the fire extinguisher from the garage, in case our plan went awry.

We looked at each other, gritted our teeth, and then tossed the first match into the can. Nothing. Then a second. Nothing. The third match caught. The contents started to smoke, and a fire blazed.

There was a loud pop. Alex and I jumped back, and a cascade of pops sounded like fireworks. Shells and egg parts burst inside the metal can. The smell of the burning eggs filled my mother's backyard with the stench of sulfur.

We plugged our noses and watched smoke and flames fill the air. Soon, the fire extinguished on its own. Once the smoke subsided, we peered inside the trash can. Only four of the eggs had burned. Two remained unscathed. We lit the contents again, and stared as the smelly snap, crackle, and pop show continued. We watched until everything burned to ashes.

"Hey, Alex, did Vladimir say anything bad about the eggs exploding? They definitely erupted. Is that the same as breaking or cracking?"

"There's no other way to destroy them." Alex's words fell flat, not convinced we had accomplished what Vladimir asked. We cleaned up the mess, and then we both took a long nap.

After six more sessions of Vladimir's post chicken-egg craziness, no more of my symptoms improved. My breasts still felt better, but my heart and all the rest of my symptoms remained the same.

The entire fertile-chicken-egg escapade was a bust, literally. The financial strain and long drives were strenuous. I didn't regret the time, effort, or the over $2,000 I had spent on this eccentric, egg-loving Russian, and felt grateful for what Vladimir had done, but I needed to make a decision.

I never saw Vladimir again.

chapter twenty-one

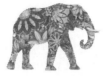

A LITTLE HELP
FROM MY FRIENDS

APRIL 2005 – SAN DIEGO

I leaned back on the small tan couch in my apartment after stacking a pile of paperwork on the coffee table in front of me. Crows squawked outside the window. An airplane flew overhead, and my heart thumped to its unique and erratic rhythm.

"Well, that's it, Bruno," I said to my new feline pal, "I'm officially unemployed." Bruno had a white-and-tangerine coat, weighed twenty-two pounds, and was ten years old. His robust body pressed against my legs, and his roaring purr resonated throughout the room.

Not long after Riley died, a few friends moved my belongings into an apartment upstairs with a secured balcony, inaccessible to coyotes or other predatory creatures. I adopted Bruno from a no-kill shelter, not to replace Riley, since nothing ever could, but to provide company for my other cat, Duke, and to me.

Meow Town was a private shelter managed and funded by a French woman named Jenée. She had a few volunteers, but never enough to attend to all the animals in need, especially since Jenée never turned any felines away, no matter what their circumstances. I recalled the first time I had ever been there.

"I've got a surprise for you," Alex said.

"What is it?"

"You'll have to come with me to find out."

I grinned. "You mean *now*?"

Alex gestured with his hand. "Unless you've got something better to do this afternoon."

We arrived at the end of a dirt road on top of a hill that ended at a private, steep driveway. Eight large wired enclosures covered the lot. Alex helped me walk to the first cage. I peered inside and saw countless cats roaming around. I felt sadness and joy.

"I found this place on the Internet," he said, looking around at the few acres of land. "I know how much you miss Riley, and how much you love cats and volunteer work, so I thought we could help out a little and get you out of the house."

"Volunteer? You know I'm not strong enough to do anything. All I could do is sit on the ground and pet them."

Alex smiled. "Exactly. I spoke with the owner. She knows your condition. She said most of the cats just want someone to love them. You can do that, right?"

I felt overwhelmed with delight to be needed again. It filled me with a new sense of purpose. I could help others. I mattered, and I wanted these felines to know that they mattered too.

"Oh, Alex, this is wonderful." I reached out to hug him.

He hugged me back.

Every Sunday we went to Meow Town, making it a ritual. Alex helped me get positioned on a chair or cushion inside the cage while he cleaned water and food bowls, and scooped litter boxes. As I sat, at least thirty cats took turns rubbing up and down against my legs, back, and feet, begging for attention. I brushed and petted them for as long as they wanted. I tried to make it to each cage on every visit, but sometimes I felt too fatigued to make the entire rounds. All the cats had wonderful personalities and fun names like Galileo, Lord Byron, Marmalade, and Sunny. I wanted to take them all with me and give them a permanent home, but I could only manage one in addition to Ducatti.

"How do I pick one from all these hundreds of cats?" I asked Alex. We stood inside one of the cages, watching cats eat, bathe, and sleep. "It doesn't seem fair that only one of them gets a home and the others don't. I can't choose."

Bruno strutted down from a perch, his rotund white tummy swaying as he walked to the food bowl. He was the tallest and biggest cat I had ever seen, and something about him made me smile. He had never lived outside of a shelter, and was already ten years old. Within a week, after an examination and a trip to the groomer for a much-needed bath and pedicure, Bruno became my newest companion.

He had asthma, severe gingivitis, and a crumpled ear from a hematoma that required continual medical attention, but to me, he was perfect. Some people mentioned I didn't need the added responsibility, since I couldn't care well for myself. I smiled knowing that the unconditional love from my felines was one of the reasons I stayed sane. They healed me more than anything else.

I stroked Bruno's head and ears and continued my one-sided conversation. "My boss was kind enough to hold my job for so long, wasn't she? Everyone thought I'd be better by now and back to work." I shifted my attention toward Duke who lay upside down with his front paws folded over. "I can't believe I've been ill for a year now." I continued petting Bruno's short, coarse fur. "Don't worry, boys, I'm going to find out why I'm sick, then get better and find a new job. We have to keep positive."

That night, Alex worked late. He often worked fourteen-hour days, most weeks seven days. I hardly saw him, and when I did, he had his laptop or Blackberry on. I hated seeing him work so hard. I could see how tired and aggravated he was, but he always told me he was thankful to have a job.

I celebrated my one-year anniversary of being ill by consuming a can of tomato soup and a glass of ice water with a slice of lime. As I sipped my soup, I watched my cats nap in the goofiest of positions, their expressions full of contentment. How I longed to feel that type of comfort.

Despite what I told them, I couldn't help but worry about my predicament. The reality of my situation troubled me. I was no closer to getting a diagnosis than a year ago, and I had no job. I stressed about money.

I got a roommate to help with expenses, a quiet and kind Korean guy named Dae-Hyun who worked as an engineer. Having a stranger in my house while I was sick felt overwhelming and difficult, but I needed the money. I sold some of my furniture and exhausted my savings to keep up with my bills. I also applied for and started receiving disability.

Alex, my mother, and my grandfather gifted me money whenever they could to help pay my expenses. My sister even sent me a check with a simple note that read, "Use this for whatever you need." I was so grateful for their support. I was good at giving, but had never been good at receiving. But the desperation of my situation, both financially and physically, left me wondering what my future would bring. Would I ever work again?

The phone rang. It was Bruce. He usually called me about once a week to check in on me. He also often made the long drive from Ramona to get me out of my apartment and take me to lunch. I set the phone on my chest and felt my heart pounding.

"How you feeling, Cherie?" Bruce's New York accent was dim, and his voice sounded tentative yet hopeful. "I thought we could have lunch again next week."

"I'll have to check my appointments. It all depends on how I feel." I had noticed a cycle with my illness. Horrible days filled with unrelenting pain, and other days when the symptoms felt manageable, and I could get out of the house, walk to the end of the street, go to the beach and watch the birds, or attempt some laundry or light cleaning. Yet often when I attempted such tasks, my symptoms intensified and I would end up worse. I had to learn to manage the limited energy and strength I had.

"Oh, Cherie. What am I going to do with you?" He sighed. "You need to get better."

A couple of days later, I met my friend Jocelyn for lunch after one of my doctor appointments. We had met through beach volleyball.

"It's good to see you out of the house, Cherie." Jocelyn pushed her bright, blond hair back from her beautiful tanned face, then sipped her raspberry iced tea. Tall, slender, always well dressed, and a pleasure to call my friend, Jocelyn and I enjoyed our conversations. Our time together was a pleasant distraction. She added, "And you're able to drive again."

"Yeah, sometimes, but it's tough. I only go short distances. I have so many appointments. I see a chiropractor, acupuncturist, massage therapist, homeopath, osteopath, nutritionist, and several specialists. I finally have a new primary doctor. It's like starting from scratch with each new person I see. I'm exhausted on top of being exhausted." I held my head up with my hand, my elbow resting on the table, my breathing forced.

I thought about my new primary doctor, Dr. Universe (who had replaced Dr. Loveless). She was in high demand because she was caring, knowledgeable, a superb listener, and spent quality time with each patient. No matter how many tests came back negative, or new symptoms emerged without explanation, she never gave up on me or thought I was making it up. Instead, she was encouraging, optimistic, and compassionate.

She believed in treating the whole person: mind, body, and spirit. I wasn't still certain about the idea of a higher power, but because of my interactions with Dr. Universe, the spiritual side of me blossomed. I began to believe in a larger purpose. No dogma, no name, no specific affiliation, simply the existence of a universal energy connecting all beings.

One of the first things she told me was, "If you were meant to die, you would have already. You've certainly had several opportunities. You're meant to be here, Cherie."

A waiter dropped a glass on the restaurant floor, and the loud crashing sound brought me back to the moment. I continued, "And it's all so expensive since my insurance says all the holistic/alternative treatments I am doing are experimental, but no traditional M.D. knows what to do with me. I've spent over $25,000 just for medical in the past year, not including what insurance has paid, which is far more."

I thought about some of the other remarkable and caring healers I employed to help me deal with my extreme set of symptoms, including Dr. Zen, an M.D. turned acupuncturist from Peru, whose mere presence made me feel calmer, and Dr. Wellness, a chiropractor who was knowledgeable not only about her field of specialty, but also nutrition, supplements, and a host of other healing modalities.

"It's no wonder so many people file for bankruptcy from medical expenses," Jocelyn said.

"It's awful."

"How's the roommate working out?"

"It's difficult being sick and having a roommate, especially someone I don't know. He's nice though. I'd prefer my own space, I just can't afford it."

The waitress placed two gigantic salads in front of us. I picked up my fork with my right hand, continuing the custom I learned in Africa, a habit I was consciously and unreasonably afraid to break. I could no longer tuck my left hand underneath my legs; I needed it to support my neck and head.

While Jocelyn spoke, uneasiness crept from my stomach to my throat. It couldn't have been the food, because I hadn't even taken a bite. I often had unusual symptoms flare up without warning. I braced myself for the unknown and moved my left hand from around my neck. Suddenly my head felt as if it were swinging in circles—a tether ball beaten by an unruly child.

I rubbed my temples.

My temples feel larger. Oh no, now my head is deformed, or is this the way it has always been? I don't remember any teacher in school ever instructing me how my head is supposed to feel. How am I supposed to know what is normal?

Jocelyn continued talking, unaware of my inner dialogue. I caught snatches of what she was saying, but my thoughts drifted back to the piercing pangs.

I tried to maintain social graces, nodding and forcing my eyes open long enough to make eye contact, but I couldn't concentrate. I needed to go home and rest.

"What do you think?" Jocelyn shoved a colossal piece of spinach into her mouth.

I had no idea what she had been talking about. I stammered, "Well, I'm not sure."

"Exactly," Jocelyn said. "No one's sure these days."

What exactly was I ambivalent about? How was my answer adequate? My throbbing headache faded as I drank some chilled water and my stomach digested the few bites of food I had taken.

I melted back into the booth, believing I could make it through the meal without causing a scene, but I knew the next onslaught of symptoms was waiting around the corner, ready to strike.

As Jocelyn continued her soliloquy of rhetorical questions, I nodded and returned to the unanswerable queries bombarding me.

The muscles around the base of my head stiffened again. Heat surrounded my skull. *Why weren't we taught that dreadful things can happen to us? What's the point of suffering? Does it make us stronger, or appreciate life? Have I become a slave to this unidentified illness? Will I ever be able to remove these shackles?* I groaned.

"You okay?"

I studied her tan, healthy-looking face. "I'm sorry, Jocelyn. I'm not."

"Was it something I said?"

"Of course not. It's just so painful. The emergency still exists. I try to remain strong, but it's so hard, not knowing why or when, if ever, this suffering is going to end."

Jocelyn set her fork on the table. "I'm so sorry, Cherie. I have no idea how hard it's been for you. I don't think anyone does."

"I've lost many friends because of this illness. I don't call any of my friends because I feel so horrible, and when I finally build up the strength to go out, like today with you, I fake how I feel and struggle to maintain my composure. I try to stay positive, but mostly I want to cry."

Jocelyn frowned. Her not saying anything meant the most to me. She understood I just needed someone to listen, someone who wasn't trying to fix me.

"Thanks for being here for me."

"Of course, Cherie. And hey, one day I may need you. You'll be there for me, right?"

"Absolutely. Anytime, for anything."

chapter twenty-two

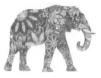

A TWIST OF...

SEPTEMBER 2005 – SAN DIEGO

I sat on a metal green bench at Lindbergh Field. Endless streams of people hurried past. Some moving quickly and purposefully, others meandering as if they had time to waste. Fluorescent lights, beeps, background music, people talking, perfumes and deodorants bombarded my neurological system.

I wanted to go home, but I couldn't. For the first time since my illness began a year and a half ago, I needed to get on a plane.

"Did someone order a wheelchair?" an airport attendant called out, looking around.

I waved to him. "I did."

He pushed the wheelchair next to the bench. The navy-blue seat was ripped, the wheels wobbly.

The attendant locked it in place, and Alex lifted me into it.

The attendant pushed down the foot rests and placed my feet upon them. "You comfortable, miss?"

"Fine, thanks. I'm flying on Southwest to Phoenix, gate eleven."

"You're not flying today, sir?" he asked Alex.

"No. But I have a pass to escort her through to the gate."

"All right then." The attendant pushed me through swarms of people, calling out for everyone to give way, drawing attention to our small convoy of three. As people parted and walked past me, they stared, their gazes confused and pensive, as if trying to determine what led me to need the wheelchair. I wondered the same.

Alex walked alongside as we maneuvered through the airport security line to a special area for people requiring extra assistance. People watched me hobble through security, held up by Alex's muscular and comforting arms. My legs shook. I had never been scared to travel before.

After a difficult goodbye, the attendant wheeled me down the ramp to the plane and helped me to my seat in the first row. At nearly the same time, another passenger arrived in a wheelchair. In his forties with a thin build and pale complexion, he hobbled to his seat beside me. We exchanged glances and smiled cordially.

Just as I wondered why he needed a wheelchair, he said, "Hi, I'm Alan. I have MS, if you're curious. What about you?"

"I—" I stumbled and couldn't conjure up the right words. "I'm sorry to hear that."

"No worries. Just thought since we're both in similar shoes, we'd be open about it instead of sitting here guessing the whole flight. So, you going to tell me?"

"I wish I could, Alan. I really do."

My mother flew in from L.A. and met me at the Phoenix airport. Since Alex was busy with work, she volunteered to spend the week with me while I saw a specialist.

On the second day, we walked arm in arm, my mother helping me into our motel room. "Why do people choose to live out here?" I wiped the sweat off my face. "It's 115 degrees." The relentless September heat of Arizona penetrated my every cell. I became even more wilted than before, like a forgotten piece of lettuce in the back of a refrigerator.

My mom shook her head. "I don't know, but at least there's air conditioning."

We plopped down on our respective lumpy beds. It had been a long and tiring two days undergoing multiple tests and examinations requested by this new physician. I began drifting off to sleep.

"Cherie, wake up." My mom's voice sounded nurturing, like when I was a child and she tried to wake me with ease in time for school. "Your cell phone's ringing."

I grabbed my phone off the nightstand. "Hello?"

"This is Dr. Nurture," one of the newest doctors I employed, a specialist in women's health issues, regenerative care, and radiology. "I know you're in Arizona seeing a specialist, but I didn't think you would want to wait to hear the news."

I pictured her bleached blond hair, long face, and kind hazel eyes. "You have my test results?"

"You tested off the charts for Epstein Barr."

"Epstein Barr?"

"A common virus present in about ninety percent of adults, but in some people it leads to more serious autoimmune challenges. Your numbers are staggering. I've never seen numbers this high before. Honestly, I don't know how you're walking around."

Tears filled my eyes. After a year and a half of searching, my heart condition was the only positive test result I had had besides fibromyalgia and chronic fatigue syndrome, which were still just symptoms. Epstein Barr joined the list.

"It explains why you're so exhausted."

I sat back on the bed while a complex stream of emotions flooded me: relief, grief, surprise.

My mother saw me sobbing and smiling. She walked over and put her hand on my shoulder. "You okay?"

I nodded, still crying, still beaming. After a few seconds, I gained some composure, "What about my other symptoms?" I asked the doctor.

"This doesn't explain those, but it's a start."

"What can I do to get rid of it?"

"There's no way to treat it. It stays in your cells, but you can become stronger over time, and it can become dormant. Rest is the most important thing."

My heart rate accelerated. I felt hot and knew red splotches were forming on my neck. "I've been resting for almost a year and a half. Isn't there anything else we can do?"

"There are some holistic remedies we can try to help with your compromised immune system. I'll get a protocol set up for when you get back. Take care, and get some rest. You need it."

My mom handed me a tissue from her purse. "What is it, Cherie?"

"That new doctor found something wrong with me. I have Epstein Barr. I'm not crazy."

My mom hugged me. "Of course you're not crazy."

"I bet it sounds strange that I'm excited to have something wrong with me."

"No, it doesn't. And all of those tests you took the past two days at this specialist's office, I bet they'll show something too."

"I hope so."

My spirits lifted. I now had one more piece to my puzzle, but there had to be something more. I needed to keep searching.

For the third consecutive day, my mother drove us from the motel to Dr. Integrative's office, a single-story tan building flanked by palm trees and rock gardens. He specialized in helping patients with rare and difficult-to-diagnose illnesses. He came recommended by one of Alex's friends who lived in Arizona.

Dr. Integrative blended conventional and alternative philosophies of medical practice while providing compassionate, individualized care. Like most of the doctors, healers, and specialists who took the time to see me and do a myriad of tests, he did not take insurance. My medical bills soared, but there was no choice.

Dr. Integrative entered the reception area and called out my name. His white hair and clean-shaven face both shone under the halogen lights. He moved with grace like a dancer, almost gliding over to me with an odd-but-happy expression on his face. In front of everyone in the waiting room, he took my hands in his and said, "I have what I hope you will consider good news. You tested positive for Lyme disease."

I looked at his face, wrinkled and serious with a tiny smirk. His eyes glistened with what felt like hope. I squeezed his hands and stood motionless, as if I had fallen prey to Medusa's mythical gaze and was now a statue of stone.

"Really?" my mom said.

"The urine test we sent to a special lab came back unequivocally positive. I even had them repeat the test three times while diluting your sample to make sure. Cherie, you have Lyme. Come on, let's talk about this." He guided us back to his office.

As we walked along the corridor, I saw patients hooked up to IVs, concoctions of solutions he used to treat cancer patients who did not respond to chemotherapy. Nurses moved from room to room, carrying charts, trays, vials, and cups.

"In here." Dr. Integrative motioned us into his office and closed the door. We all sat. My hands trembled. Lyme disease. Ticks, parasites, blood. My blood was tainted.

I said nothing. I had waited so long to find out what ailed me. Now I had two positive test results in two days.

"I hope I didn't alarm you. I mean what I said. I consider this good news," he said in a reassuring tone.

I took a couple of deep breaths before speaking. "It may sound strange, but I believe the one part I've missed out on all this time is the relief of having some kind of solid diagnosis. Now that I have one, I don't know what to say."

"That doesn't sound strange at all." Dr. Integrative rocked back in his chair. "I see many patients who don't know where else to turn. They end up in my office. I have to pick up the pieces where the other doctors left off and have not ventured any further. In several cases, the insurance companies dictate which tests and treatments patients get, so it's often not the doctor's fault. It's a failure of mainstream medicine. I consider it a privilege to help those like you in need."

My mother asked, "Doctor, what exactly is Lyme?"

"A bacterial disease transmitted by ticks."

"Ticks? When were you around ticks, Cherie?"

I shook my head, trying to think of a time I had ever seen a tick. I couldn't recall any.

"A lot of people never know they've been bitten," the doctor said. "It's often a silent transmission. It's also a non-discriminating disease that affects all parts of the body and can cause numerous debilitating symptoms that vary from person to person. It can mimic several other illnesses, but if it's caught early, it can be treated by antibiotics. If left undiagnosed, like in your case, it can cause severe damage."

"What do I do now?"

"There are several approaches. We need to get you set up with a practitioner you trust back home who can administer the protocol I'm about to propose."

I thought of Dr. Nurture, and a doctor I had recently met named Dr. Open, and how they were both medical doctors who teetered on the more holistic approach to healing. They would be the first ones I would contact. "What about the Epstein Barr?"

Dr. Integrative smiled and scratched his head, leaving a tuft of white hair sticking straight up in the air. "We'll work to strengthen your immune system too. Now, let's get started."

I arrived back in San Diego on a dry, warm, gusty day. Santa Ana winds swept over the coastline, parching my lips and skin. I clung to Alex as we sat on the couch embracing each other. "It's good to be home."

Exhausted from five days of extreme heat, donating almost thirty vials of blood, and undergoing a number of unusual tests, I could hardly stay awake. As we cuddled, Alex flipped through television stations, stopping on an episode of Seinfeld.

"Have you seen this one?" he asked.

"Which one is it?"

"Elaine's planning a baby shower at Jerry's apartment."

"I don't remember." My eyelids closed.

A few moments later, Alex sat up straight and tapped me in the shoulder. "CK, did you hear that?"

I opened my eyes. "Huh, no, what?"

"The reason Elaine is using Jerry's apartment for the baby shower is because her roommate has Epstein Barr and Lyme disease!"

I sat up at attention, stared at the screen. "Whoa. What are the odds?" I asked.

"It seems par for the course for you."

A few days after my newest diagnosis, I caught this rerun on television. I had, as Elaine so eloquently put it, "Epstein Barr with a twist of Lyme disease." Could this be it? Could it be this simple?

Either way, I felt delighted to know what was wrong with me, but after seeing a couple of doctors to confirm my diagnosis, not everyone believed me, and not all of the pieces fit. I took two more Lyme tests while back in San Diego. Both came back negative. The doctors in San Diego said the one positive lab test wasn't credible.

Hopelessness and doubt crept in. And once again, I felt lost. Was it really Lyme? Or was there something else?

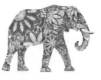

chapter twenty-three

To Pee or Not to Pee

MAY 2006 – SAN DIEGO

JOURNAL ENTRY

Being ill is difficult enough without all of the logisti-
cal problems patients have to deal with, including piles
of medical paperwork, lab mishaps, poorly organized
medical offices, inept people, and of course, the post
office. What has happened to a lot of my mail? In one
instance, I didn't know I had an outstanding bill until
I received an impolite telephone call from a collection
agency accusing me of not paying, and threatening me if
I didn't. I attempted to explain I had no idea what bill
she was referring to, and if she would please send me a
copy I would investigate the charges and pay if it was
a legitimate charge. I guess she had heard every excuse
before and refused to listen. She was curt and rude. I was
presumed guilty.

I closed my journal and hobbled outside to check my mail. It felt
good to vent, even if it was only on paper. The details of my illness
often felt like mountains I carried on my back. I felt like a work mule
inching its way up an endless, hot, rock-strewn road carrying an over-
weight, flatulent, unappreciative tourist who kept digging his cheap
cowboy boots into my ribs. I continued to work hard trying to cure
myself. Alex believed I overachieved at it, but what else could I do?

Returning to my apartment, I brought back a stack of new medical bills, a mound of junk mail, and a package I had been waiting for, another Lyme test. For the past six months, I had weathered vitamin IV treatments given by Dr. Open and Dr. Nurture, taken several supplements and minerals, foul tasting herbs, homeopathy, and received injections to treat the suspected Lyme disease. I tried everything anyone suggested might help for Lyme. Nothing helped. In fact, most of the treatments made my symptoms worse.

This was my fifth time testing for Lyme, but it was a new type of test. Three tests had come back negative. The only one that had come back positive was the first one in Phoenix.

In search of a doctor to support me in treatments since my diagnosis in Arizona, many questioned the accuracy of the original test and doubted I ever had Lyme. A few even implied I had concocted the story.

One who was especially adamant about his position on Lyme disease, Dr. Know-It-All, was a graduate of Yale Medical School. He was a successful rheumatologist in San Diego who dealt primarily with autoimmune diseases, as well as clinical problems involving the joints, muscles, and connective tissue.

He was always overbooked, and I had to wait weeks to get a fifteen-minute consultation.

"You don't have Lyme disease," Dr. Know-It-All said, leaning against the counter across from me. I noticed his clean-shaven, smooth complexion, and an aura about him that said, "I was prom king, sat at the cool kids table, and was voted mostly likely to succeed."

I was in my normal position: lying on the examination table, holding my neck while Alex held my hand.

"How can you be so sure?" Alex said. "The specialist in Phoenix said—"

"I'm from Connecticut, where Lyme disease was first discovered. There's no Lyme disease in California." Dr. Know-It-All tapped the end of his pen on the counter.

"Not one case in the whole state?" Alex asked.

Before he could answer, I said, "I've also traveled all over the United States and to more than forty countries. Even if you don't think I got it in California, maybe..."

Dr. Know-It-All shook his head. "It doesn't matter. There's no such thing as chronic Lyme."

We left, dumbfounded by this man. Dr. Integrative in Phoenix had been so certain. Did I really have Lyme? I needed to find out.

I opened the package, rationalizing that this new test would be worth all $195. It would show me whether I had Lyme or not, and therefore, dictate what I would do next.

It was a three-day urine test. The instructions stated that the samples had to be sent Federal Express on the third day. The fourth day pick-up was a risk because the samples needed to be "fresh," as if someone were going to drink them or use them to fertilize their garden. They also had to be shipped on either Monday, Tuesday, or Wednesday at the latest to ensure they arrived by Friday, since the lab was not open on Saturday.

Saturday was the best day to start my collections. I would call FedEx Monday morning so the samples would be at the lab by Wednesday, plenty of time before the Friday deadline.

I woke up Saturday morning with my period. It had arrived five days early. There was no mention of avoiding these days in the instructions. It was either not important, they forgot to mention it, or, the writer was a man. The following weekend I woke up again early on Saturday and proceeded with the urine collection. Nothing like the robust smell of urine first thing in the morning. Although I couldn't do many things, at least I could still pee on my own. Ah, the simple pleasures in life.

By Sunday evening, I had completed two of the samples and stored them in a brown paper bag in the back of my refrigerator on a fortress of paper towels in an attempt to separate them from my food. In a thick black pen, I wrote on the bag, "Do not touch or drink," like I would ever make that mistake.

I called FedEx to schedule a pick-up.

"Tomorrow's Memorial Day," the representative said. "No pick-ups can be scheduled."

Crap.

"What about Tuesday? Can I schedule a pick-up for that morning?" Tuesday would be the fourth and last day I could ship my samples since I had started on Saturday.

"We can't do that," the representative said.

"Why not?"

"Because of the holiday weekend, the station near your home may be too busy, so we can't schedule it."

I explained my predicament.

With a snippy tone, she said, "You should have been more prepared and thought about the holiday and planned better."

My face felt hot. I took a couple of shallow breaths. "Please, what can I do to ensure this package gets picked up on Tuesday?"

"Call FedEx on Tuesday morning."

"I can call them on Tuesday morning to get it picked up on Tuesday morning?"

"No, you can call Tuesday morning and a representative will help you schedule then."

"You can't help me now?"

"Correct."

I sighed. "Okay. Thanks for everything."

Shaking from adrenaline, I had an urge to run ten miles to release my aggression, but I couldn't. My running days were over. I closed my eyes and pictured myself fit and sturdy, sprinting along the sand, my stride long and my arms smoothly moving by my sides. I longed to have that freedom again.

But even as bad as my life felt, I knew things could be worse.

chapter twenty-four

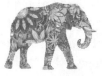

POSITIVELY NEGATIVE

JUNE 2006 – SAN DIEGO

The phone rang. It was Bruce.

"Hey, I've been thinking about you," I said, excited to talk with him. "I've left you a few messages."

"Sorry about that. I've been busy."

"Well, I miss you."

"I miss you too, Cherie."

"I'm feeling decent this week. I'd love to see you for lunch if you can."

A few seconds passed with only silence, and then I heard Bruce clear his throat. "Ah, that's not going to happen."

"Okay, what about next week?"

"Cherie, I've got something to tell you."

Now I was silent.

"I've got cancer."

A burning pain encompassed my eyes, and tightness gripped my stomach.

"It's metastasized. In my organs. We caught it late. I'm having surgery this week. Then chemo."

"Oh God, no."

He didn't say anything more. I fumbled to find words. "I'm so sorry, Bruce."

"Yeah, me too."

I wiped tears from my cheeks. "Can I come see you?"

"Nah. You focus on your health."

"But I want to. Please? And I'm going to be here for you, just like you've been for me. We'll get through this."

"You just take care of yourself, Cherie. Promise?"

More tears pooled in my eyes. "I promise."

Bruce survived the surgery that removed the largest of his tumors. He then started chemo. I visited him when able, although it was often weeks in between my visits because of my symptoms. He was strong. And I tried to be strong for him and his wife, Rebecca.

For weeks I continued to shed tears for Bruce, for my persistent ailments, and the exhaustion of navigating the medical system. Paperwork, phone calls, waiting rooms, and regulations meant to protect me kept getting in my way. I received a generic lab report concerning my urine analysis. No results were listed, only confirmation that the samples were received and my check cashed.

I took initiative and called the lab. The results had been sent to Dr. Open, who had not received them.

"I can't do that," the lab representative said, vexation filtering through the receiver.

"But I'm the patient. That's my urine, and I paid for the test. Can you please tell me if they were negative or positive? I can discuss the rest with the doctor."

"We can't tell you. It's against the law."

"I'm giving you permission. You can quote me, tape record this conversation, whatever." I felt the muscles around my jaw tighten. I had heard this speech before from a different lab, months ago. I hoped she would sense my urgency and comply.

"We can only release the results to the referring physician."

"Tell me—don't you think the system's crazy? You're not the patient, doctor, or a nurse and you know my results. How unfair is that?"

No matter what I said, the person on the other end of the phone would never tell me, but I still needed to try.

"All I can do is fax something to your doctor asking for his signature. He has to fax it back, and then I can fax him the results, then he can call you and give you the results."

"But I'm talking with you right now, and you have them in front of you. You would be doing me an enormous favor."

"Sorry, I can't. It's—"

"I know, against the law. HIPPA regulations. What an appropriate name. Hypocritical, hippopotamus, whatever."

"Is there anything else I can do for you?" She sounded more than annoyed.

"Besides giving me the results?"

"Yes, besides that."

"I guess not."

Dr. Open was a kind and caring man with a thick Midwestern accent and often wore cowboy boots and a bolo tie. He said he would help in whatever way he could. So, I called the lab once again.

"Hello, this is Sally, may I help you?"

"Yes, hello. I called a few minutes ago, and I spoke with you about my Lyme test."

"Yes, I remember." She sounded amazed that I had the audacity to call back.

I felt ashamed of my earlier behavior. "Ah, well," I cleared my throat. "I spoke with my doctor. He said fax over the paper."

"I'll do it now."

"Thanks for your help." I half wondered why she didn't ask if there was anything else she could help me with.

At 1 p.m. I called Dr. Open. He was busy with a patient and said he would call when he finished. I waited by the phone all day like a crazed teenage girl waiting to hear from her latest crush. At almost 9:30 p.m. the phone rang.

"Hello there, young lady."

"Hi, Dr. Open."

"I have the test results. They were all negative."

"All three of them?"

"Yes. Negative, negative, negative. With all of the IV therapy you've been doing for the Lyme, there may not be any particles in your urine." His tone attempted to be reassuring, but it wasn't.

"Maybe the test would have been different if I had taken it back in September before all of these treatments?"

"Perhaps."

"I'm not sure what this means."

"It's tough to know." He sounded tired and reluctant to talk.

"Thanks for all your help. I appreciate it."

I hung up the phone, collapsed onto the floor, and stared at the ceiling. Alex came and sat next to me. Two tears slalomed down the sides of my face and dripped into my ears. I grimaced and reached for his hand.

"I'm sorry, hon." His voice sounded sensitive and soft.

I cried for the indignity, the longing to know and understand the reason or reasons behind my illness, and the cruel disease in my blood, perhaps hiding in my tissues. Was it something we could ever find? Did modern medical science even have a name for it? Maybe the vagueness regarding my sickness was meant to persist, for some greater good, a greater good I could not foresee.

Nonsense.

The not knowing steadily devoured my spirit. Maybe my pursuit to identify what ailed me was fruitless. Maybe Dr. Loveless was right. Maybe I was insane, and maybe I was too crazy to know it.

chapter twenty-five

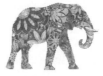

MOVING ON AND MOVING UP

NOVEMBER 2006 – SAN DIEGO

My cell phone rang. The display read "Bruce calling." I grinned with excitement. I hadn't heard from him in two weeks. It wasn't like him not to return calls.

"Hey," I answered, "I've been worried about you. How have you—"

"Cherie, Rebecca here. I couldn't find your number then I remembered it was programmed into Bruce's phone."

"Oh hey, Rebecca." I was happy to hear from her for a brief moment, then I experienced a tsunami of foreboding building inside me. "I've been trying to get in touch with you guys. What's going on?"

"I checked Bruce into San Diego Hospice a few days ago. His pain was so bad. I couldn't take care of him anymore."

I raised my hand against my cheek to halt the tears trickling down my face. It had all happened so fast. Was he really dying?

She cleared her throat. "This may sound strange, and I don't know if I believe in this kind of stuff, but the doctors are amazed he's still alive. There's a medium trying to connect with Bruce to help him pass over. He's on so much morphine it's difficult to communicate. He's hallucinating, mumbling. She believes he said goodbye to me and his family, but is holding on because he hasn't had a chance to say goodbye to you. I wouldn't ask if it wasn't important. I know you have a lot going on. We weren't going to let friends come by since we thought it would be too much, but the medium feels there's a woman besides me who he needs to connect with before he passes. I know how close the two of you are. Maybe if you spend time with him, he'll be able to let go."

I inhaled, filling my lungs with what felt like heavy black clouds of sorrow.

"Of course, Rebecca. I'll leave right now."

"Thank you. It's on Third Street."

I hung up and broke into hysterics, crying, searching for a place on the floor to sit amongst the poop and blood-stained rugs from Ducatti who had recently had colon-rectal pull-through surgery to remove obstructing tumors and half of his colon, an emergency procedure that had saved his life. Ducatti was my baby, my dearest companion, who now needed twenty-four-hour care. He could no longer control his bowel movements. Poop covered the floor, bedspread, walls, and of course, me and Alex. We often woke with poop next to our faces where Ducatti had slept. It gave a whole new meaning to unconditional love. We alternated caring for him in my bedroom, but the stress from caring for and constantly cleaning him, us, and the mounds of laundry made me even feebler, and my ability to perform daily tasks even harder.

San Diego Hospice was at least thirty miles away, with rush-hour traffic, a minimum one-hour drive. Sleep-deprived, my muscles shook, and I knew I shouldn't be in a car, let alone driving one, but this was my chance to do something that mattered for Bruce, Rebecca, his family, and me.

I forced myself up from the floor, grabbed my keys and closest pair of shoes. I stumbled down the stairs, and climbed into the car.

My vision hazy from tears, all I could see was brake lights and exhaust in both directions. I strained to see the speedometer. Fifteen miles an hour. I wanted to race around the other cars.

What if he died before I got there?

I wasn't familiar with southern San Diego, I was always a North County girl. After an hour navigating three different highways, I exited the freeway and found my way, remembering years before when I had run a marathon there.

I turned on the radio to soothe my racing thoughts. The delicate, haunting voice of Sarah McLachlan sang her song, *I Will Remember You*.

Lost in my thoughts, I ran a stop sign then immediately pulled over, surprised by my recklessness.

Crap, Cherie.

I thought of a scene from the movie *Airplane*, when a passenger freaked out because they had lost both pilots. A line of people waited to shake her, slap her, and tell her to "Get a hold of yourself."

I turned up the volume.

As the melancholic tune caressed my ears, I understood that I needed Bruce more than he needed me. It had always been so throughout our friendship and illnesses. The times I visited him during his chemo, after his surgeries, his radiant smile and brilliant intellect saved me from myself. Could I help him now?

The cheerless song finished, and I re-entered the city streets. I saw Third Street and pulled into the hospice parking lot, where I spotted Rebecca pacing near several parked cars.

I rolled down my window to greet her, but before I could think of what to say, she sobbed, "I can't believe this. I don't need this right now."

"What's wrong?"

"My sister locked my keys in the car," she shrieked.

"I'll help, let me park." I had no idea how I could assist other than call a tow truck. I parked, walked over to Rebecca, and hugged her.

She was not in the mood for softness. She needed to unleash built-up hostility and rage. She pulled away from me and shouted, "I'm so pissed off!"

How again was it I was going to help?

"I'm sorry, Cherie. It's been a hard night. We've got a tow truck on its way. I'm just frustrated, overwhelmed, and frankly, mad, but thank you for coming."

"I'm so glad you called. I want to help. Can I see him?"

She spoke as we walked to the back entrance of the single-story building. "I've been with him every day, and I've watched his decline, but for you, not having seen him in weeks..." She paused. "He doesn't look good. I want you to mentally prepare yourself, okay?"

"Okay," I whispered, then sobbed. I tried to stop my tears. Rebecca wrapped her arm around my shoulders and let me cry.

"I'm sorry," I mumbled.

"That's okay. I would rather you cry out here before we get inside."

"Me too. I'm all right now. I won't cry in front of Bruce. Let's go."

We walked down the hall and slipped into his room. Bruce lay on a hospital bed with white cotton linens, IV drips and bags of medicine streaming into his arms. I remembered how he looked when he was well, and I recalled how he looked when he was sick. But what I hadn't seen until that moment was my friend, the avid cyclist, the natural hiker, the gifted engineer, the childish tractor-driving fanatic, and the fifty-two-year-old dog-loving human as a man on the threshold of death. Until that second, I had not believed he was dying. Yet now seeing him, I knew.

His skin looked pale, limp against his bones. He had shed a lot of weight since I last saw him six weeks ago. His six-foot-four-inch frame looked angular and gaunt. His skull protruded and was almost clear to view. His eyes stayed closed, and his mouth hung open. He swayed back and forth, the strong-willed man inside the decrepit structure of bones and flesh struggling to escape.

I wanted to run and find him somewhere else. At his desk at work, on his bike, in his house, driving his truck, or even receiving chemo, but not here, not like this. Where was my friend?

I wanted it to be a mistake, the wrong room, wrong diagnosis, wrong anything. We were both going to conquer our illnesses and look back at the whole experience. But that wasn't going to happen, at least not for him.

I sat beside his bed and smiled. I wanted him to see me smile, or somehow know I was smiling. I needed courage, but inside I was frightened.

"Hi, buddy," I said in my sturdiest voice. "Rebecca called me to come see you. I'm so glad she did. I've missed you."

His response came low and guttural. I didn't understand what he had said.

"Bruce, Cherie's here to see you. And Cherie, this is Bruce's brother, Adam," Rebecca said, pointing to a man sitting on the other side of the bed. I hadn't even noticed him. He was a younger, clean-shaven, healthy version of Bruce, with the same faint New York accent.

"Nice to meet you," I said.

"You too, Cherie. I've heard good things about you from Bruce."

I smiled, not knowing what to say. I half expected Bruce to jump into the conversation, but he just moaned and rocked from side to side. Rebecca understood some of what Bruce tried to communicate.

It was impossible to know what Bruce wanted, but I felt compelled to hold on to him somehow. I reached out, touched Bruce's arm, and held his hand. His hand felt dry and bony. I gently squeezed it in mine. It stayed limp.

"I've wanted to see you so many times," I said.

"It's not your fault," Rebecca said. "I know you've tried, but with all of Bruce's appointments and visitors, and your illness..." Her words drifted off, sounding lonely and desperate. She answered for him as if he wasn't in the room, which saddened me. I wanted Bruce to say something, but she continued to speak, and Bruce did not.

I gazed at him, still smiling, and became part of the conversation without him. Adam, Rebecca, and I shared stories, and every once in a while, Rebecca would say, "Isn't that right, Bruce?" I asked him questions, even though I knew he wouldn't answer, and in some cases I knew the answer, but I wanted to include him.

Rebecca and I went to get some water, and she said words I had been both expecting and dreading.

"Adam and I are going to wait outside while you spend some alone time with him, so you can say goodbye. Come out into the hall when you're done."

How would I ever be finished saying goodbye? I didn't want to leave. I wanted to sleep on the floor and stay with him until the end, but it wasn't my place. I wasn't his wife, sister, or any other relative. I was just a friend. What right did I have to ask for more?

I went back into the room and sat once again in the chair beside his bed, taking his cold, frail hand in mine. "Hey, it's me again, Cherie."

I studied his face, trying to memorize it, to take home with me when I would be unable to see it. Although we were close and had been through so much together, we hadn't discussed our feelings for each other. Now was the time.

"I'm so sorry this happened to you, Bruce. You don't deserve this. I want you to know how much your friendship has meant to me. You were a companion and co-worker before my illness, and a constant support since I became ill. You always made me feel special, but I realize you make everyone feel that way. Your eyes, your smile, your interest when someone speaks. I love you, Bruce. I've never said it to you before, but I do. I always will."

I paused and looked down at his bony hand clenched in mine. He rocked back and forth, shaking his head, mumbling. Was he trying to tell me something? I ran into the hallway to fetch Rebecca.

We rushed back into the room and stood beside him.

"What is it, Bruce? You need something?" Rebecca asked.

He muttered and groaned.

"Ah." Rebecca grinned. "You want some ice cream? Sure. I bet your mouth's dry and that would feel good." Bruce loved ice cream. His favorite was mocha chip.

Bruce mumbled again, louder than before.

"You don't want ice cream?"

Bruce shook his head, and Rebecca understood, like a mother with her child, comprehending utterances that everyone else hears as some form of alien-speak.

"Cherie?"

Bruce nodded.

"Yes, Bruce, Cherie's here." She looked at me. "He's saying your name."

A robust sweet, warm feeling filled my chest.

Bruce grew restless. I grasped his hand, bent over and kissed him gently on the forehead, whispering, "I will always remember you." Then I walked to the door, hugged Rebecca, nodded to Adam, and headed for the neon-green exit sign.

Bruce passed away the next day with Rebecca by his side, and me, thirty miles north, praying for a miracle that would never come. When the phone rang, Rebecca gave me the news. Although not surprised, I had still hoped he would somehow be saved.

"Cherie, I want to ask you to say something at the service, if you want to."

"I would be honored."

"I'll see you Thursday then."

"Yes. And Rebecca, I'm—"

"I know. Thanks."

After Bruce's service, I sat alone on my bed, staring at the one photograph I had of him, his glasses sturdy on his face, his navy-blue flannel shirt under his corduroy sport coat, his debonair grin.

I spoke to the picture, as if he were there beside me.

"You would have liked the service. Your Bianchi bike stood at the front of the mortuary next to a handsome photograph of you. Your remains were gifted to medical science. I'm certain you did this with the hope of bringing research closer to finding a cure for the merciless cancer that took your last breath.

"I stood near your bike, the one I used to ride next to, and I spoke before your family and friends. Seventy-five people I didn't know heard the words that should have been spoken to you. There were many things I didn't say to you, but believed you understood."

Each day for the next two weeks I spoke aloud to him. My cats probably thought I was speaking to them, and as usual, they ignored me.

"I feel so much guilt. Why was I spared while you withered away? I couldn't stop it. Nobody could. It doesn't make sense. You had a diagnosis, and I don't. We should have been able to save you.

"I was the one who became sick first, and you never strayed like others did. You recognized the importance of presence. You understood the meaning of friendship. Even when you became ill and were in so much pain, when I was trying to be there for you, you were more concerned about being there for me."

One night, I had a dream of pristine skies and the eloquence of clouds, and they all led me to Bruce. It was so clear—a peaceful stream flowing through the center of my thoughts. I saw his pre-cancer face first, vibrant, and alive. He grinned at me as I called out while I waited in a long line to sign up for a beach volleyball tournament, something I once took for granted. Now, I could only dream about it.

"Bruce. It's me, Cherie."

"Hey there," he said with his charismatic smile.

"It's wonderful to see you." I stretched out my arms to greet him.

"And you." He reached out his long, well-built arms.

We hugged, a fulfilling and warm embrace that lasted for hours, then our arms lowered, and we stood next to each other, content and smiling.

"Do you want to come with me?" I asked.

"I can't." He gave me one final smile, and disappeared.

The morning after, I woke with a sense of consolation, an understanding of what that dream meant. We were headed in different directions. It was time to face this world on my own and face my illness without him.

I closed my eyes, pressing his photograph near my chest, remembering the last thing I said at his memorial service: "One day we will ride again together, unobstructed and free, and we will leave our illnesses in the dust."

chapter twenty-six

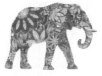

A Fond Reunion

September 2007 – Los Angeles

I met John in a trendy Santa Monica café. It had been more than thirteen years since I had seen my fellow Peace Corps volunteer. The last time we had met was in Mansa, the small capital of Luapula province in northern Zambia.

His short brown wavy hair and clear-rimmed glasses looked the same. His pale skin was adorned with a Milky Way of light freckles, and he wore a long-sleeved navy shirt and jeans. It felt like not a day had passed since I had seen him, as if part of me returned to Africa. I reflected for a moment about my time in Zambia. I no longer felt disappointed about not being able to fulfill my service, and I didn't long to go back. All I wanted was to heal.

I approached John. He glanced up from reading a book, stood to greet me, and gave me a warm, comforting hug. We sat down and he looked me over. He flashed a wide grin. "Cherie, it's really good to see you."

I grinned. "You too, John."

I was in L.A. visiting my mom, taking time off from all my doctor appointments. He was in L.A. for a series of media events to promote his memoir about being deaf and the challenges he faced living in Zambia. He mentioned me in the book, naming me Susie. He wrote, "Susie from L.A., energetic and idealistic in her sports bra, developed a puzzling and painful illness that was eventually

193

diagnosed as an infection of her diaphragm muscle lining. None of us had ever heard of such a thing."

Until just recently reading his book, I had never heard of such a thing either! Clearly, a result of the classic children's game: Telephone.

We talked about his memoir and our lives since our days in the Peace Corps. He told me of his new cochlear implants and his health challenges from surgeries. I told him all about my health.

John watched my mouth, accustomed to reading lips, even after his surgery. There's something soothing about conversing with someone who pays attention to every word.

"It must be emotionally draining for you, Cherie. I just can't imagine. How do you cope?"

"Lots of support and love." I thought about Bruce. It had been almost a year since he had died, and just recently my kitty Bruno had died too. He had developed congestive heart failure and suffered a massive blood clot in his left front leg. His ability to cuddle for long hours had given me so much comfort during many days when I was alone.

I continued. "I was also volunteering at a private animal shelter, which I loved. But I contracted toxoplasmosis, a parasitic disease common in stray felines. The doctors recommended I stop going there. It was the one part of my life where I was able to give back. Now, that's gone as well. It makes me angry."

"I'm sorry for everything you've gone through." He reached across the table and took my hand. Goose bumps covered my arms. I felt like the female lead in an inspirational made-for-TV movie.

"Thanks, John. Same goes for you." Until reading his book, I had never comprehended how much he had weathered in Zambia, just as he had never understood what had happened to me.

"Do the doctors think it all goes back to Africa?"

I wanted to talk about anything but this, like how to clean that disgusting ring around an old toilet bowl or how our eyeballs rot after we die.

I took a slow breath. "That's one theory. But no one knows. We may never know."

John sighed. "Anything I can do to help?"

I never knew how to answer this question, since I didn't know what I needed.

I shook my head and mouthed, "No, but thank you." I changed the subject. "I'm looking forward to your book signing."

"Be wonderful to have you there."

I slid my copy of his book across the table. "Sign it, will you?"

"Of course." He took the book and pulled out a pen. I excused myself to go to the restroom. When I returned, I noticed the book face down next to my purse.

John glanced at his watch. "So, I gotta get going."

"Me too. I need a nap. You wore me out." We both laughed.

John walked me out, and we hugged goodbye. Some people know how to hug, they don't hold back, and I will always cherish that about him.

We stared at each other for a few moments and parted without words. Not saying anything can mean so much. John knew that well. He walked away. I looked down at his book in my hand, opened it and read his inscription. "For Cherie—Who knows what health really is."

chapter twenty-seven

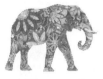

THE POWER
OF NUMBERS

OCTOBER 2008 – SAN DIEGO

Alex typed with fervor on his Blackberry at the dining room table, while I reclined on the couch, thinking about our lives. We had recently moved in together. I hoped soon I would be well and we would resume our romantic relationship. Until then, we agreed it was best to sleep in different bedrooms since I was often up most nights in pain, and he needed his sleep. Just because I suffered through the long nights didn't mean he should too. It sometimes felt lonely, but I often had my kitty Ducatti to comfort me, since, after all, he was nocturnal.

I walked over to Alex and placed a piece of paper in front of him on the table. He looked up from his Blackberry. "What's this?"

"I've been abusing my calculator."

He raised his right eyebrow.

I read the title. "What I Know: Statistics from my illness, April 2004 – October 2008."

Alex examined my lists.

What I Know, in Numbers
Alternative therapists/healers seen: 27
Blood tests (the most in one blood draw was 27 vials): Hundreds
CAT scans: 5

Counseling sessions: 49
Doctor appointments: 257
EKGs: Hundreds
Heart rate monitors worn: 5
IV treatments: 35
Loved ones who have died since I became ill: 6
Medical doctors and specialists consulted: 46
Miles driven to appointments: 12,872
MRIs: 7
Other types of tests conducted: Hundreds
Prescriptions filled: Hundreds
Remedies and supplements tried: Hundreds
Therapies tried: 41
Treatment and therapy sessions attended: 517
Ultrasounds: 10
Visits to emergency room or admitted to a hospital: 12
Vitamin injections: Hundreds
X-Rays: 19

What I Know, in Units of Time

Days I was sick: 1,710
Days I spent trying to find a diagnosis: 1,710
Days I spent trying to heal: 1,710
Days I wished I was healthy again: 1,710
Hours I contemplated giving up: Thousands
Moments I contemplated suicide: Hundreds

What I Know, in U.S. Dollars

Total amount spent on medical expenses since I became
    ill = $101,000.
Note: Total is solely what I paid and does not include amounts
    paid by insurance.

What I Still Do Not Know

Diagnosis for my illness
Cure for my illness
If there is a diagnosis
If there is a cure
What caused my illness
What, if anything, is still undiagnosed
If I will ever be healthy again

Alex looked up from the paper clenched in his hand. "Wow!"

"Staggering, isn't it? Especially if you consider that unless I find a diagnosis and cure tomorrow, these numbers will only continue to go up."

He shook his head, gave me a tender half hug, and then started typing once again.

I stared at Alex. A surge of emotion rushed through me. I felt intense love and respect, yet I also felt so alone. Our lives revolved around my illness and his work. I hated that he worked such long hours and just couldn't help but wonder if we would ever again be anything more than friends.

chapter twenty-eight

ONCE AGAIN

MAY 2009 – SAN DIEGO

JOURNAL ENTRY

You know you're having a bad week when you call 911,
the paramedics come to your house, and one of them
notices you've rearranged your furniture.

One evening while lying in bed, my heart pounding and my stomach weak from nausea, I wondered why Alex helped me. I hated being so reliant on him. I missed my independence. I longed to live without fear. And I wanted Alex to have a life, not be a nurse's aide.

I envisioned living alone, driving a car, caring for myself. Feeling free.

Those images made me smile. Then I cringed. Maybe somehow my dependence on Alex was prohibiting my healing? Maybe I relied on him too much. My meandering thoughts didn't make sense. I loved him. He loved me. We should be together.

Alex spent several hours each day conducting work on the phone. Most days I tuned out the engineering speak, but sometimes he spoke with family and friends, updating them on my status.

As I struggled to find a comfortable position in bed, I heard Alex talking on the phone with his best friend from Arizona.

"No, she's not exaggerating." Alex's voice sounded authoritative. "Trust me, I've been there. No one wants to be in the ER with someone in the bed to the left vomiting, someone in the bed to the right with diarrhea, only to have doctors come in and say they have no idea what to do with you, and then go back home again more exhausted than when you went in. This is a woman who completed higher education; trekked across the world; was incredibly fit, athletic and adventurous; was making a substantial income; and was living her life fully in ways that I admired—more so than I was ever living mine—and now she has none of that. Who wants that?"

There were a few minutes of silence, then I heard Alex speak again. "I help her because I love her. Because I am her friend. Because I can. Because the rest of society makes me angry in how they treat ill people. She's done everything anyone would or should do, in my opinion, to fix her situation. If we decided she should or should not do something, she made it happen. Period. No slipping. No whining. Minimal outward depression beyond what was reasonable for the circumstances. And even with all she has endured, she never once acted like a victim. If she can keep from falling apart mentally in addition to dealing with the physical challenges, then I can sure as heck take care of her physically and deal with the mental challenges. I feel I can make a substantive difference to someone who deserves my help, so I choose to help."

Happy, grateful tears trickled onto my pillow, the kind that release doubt, and reaffirm good in the world. I thanked the universe for Alex, and drifted off into a light slumber, clutching my chest, feeling the erratic beat of my heart.

Four hours later, when only the moon was awake to keep me company, my heart rate escalated. This time, it felt like my heart was going to explode.

"Alex!" I screamed.

Alex ran to my side. I pointed to my heart. He took my hand, felt for my pulse, and placed his head on my chest. "Oh, Cherie. It's much worse. I'm calling 911. Hang on."

202

Minutes later, two paramedics arrived, strapped me onto a mobile gurney, and hoisted me up into an ambulance. From the corner of my eye, I glimpsed my neighbors in their pajamas and robes lined up on the sidewalk, watching.

The doors of the van slammed shut. Seconds later, the ambulance barreled down the street. Alex followed in his Jeep.

The twenty-something paramedic lifted his hand toward my mouth. "These are nitrates. In case you are having a heart attack."

I opened wide. The odd chemical flavor assaulted my tongue.

"You're heart rate is 195. Just try and breathe."

I smiled. "Yes. Good idea." I took in a deep breath. I felt an intense calm. I had done this before. Many times. But this time, I wasn't scared. I was alert, aware of the power of the moment.

I surveyed my surroundings. *So, this is how I'm going to die?*

The paramedic leaned over me and said, "You're going to be okay."

My shoulders relaxed, and I smiled again. "I know. Even if I die, I'll be okay."

He furrowed his brow and stared at me like I was a few marbles shy of sane.

I was now, for the first time in all these years, truly paying attention. I closed my eyes, and let go.

chapter twenty-nine

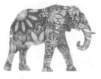

TABLE FOR ONE

AUGUST 2009 – SAN DIEGO

Bright lights covered the ceiling. I squinted. Without being able to lift my head, I looked from side to side, watching three different cardiac nurses move about. My frail body lay rigid on the cold metal operating table. My head, legs, and arms strapped down, a defibrillator, blood pressure monitor, and numerous electrodes affixed to my chest, legs, and forehead. I felt like Frankenstein's monster.

"Hello, Cherie. My name's Dr. Eager, I'm the anesthesiologist. I'm going to inject the fentanyl into your IV now. Do you have any questions before I do?"

All I could see was her tan, manicured hand holding a needle. "I want to see the cardiologist first, please."

"He's on his way."

"I'll wait. You guys can't start the heart procedure without me, right?" I grinned.

"Very well." She placed the plastic cap back on the long needle.

A few minutes later, one of the nurses leaned over me. "I also have Wolff-Parkinson-White," she said with a hint of tension. "My symptoms aren't so bad, nothing like yours, but I've been told I also need an ablation procedure. I've just been too afraid to do it, so I keep putting it off."

I strained to focus on her face, since I couldn't move my head.

Oh my goodness!

I jiggled my eyes back and forth as if to point to my body fastened to the table with large straps. "As you can see, I've made the decision to go through with it." Still stunned from her comment, I continued, "I guess you can watch how things go with me, and then make a more informed decision?"

She smiled, seeming a bit relieved at my suggestion. "I guess you're right."

Isn't she supposed to be the one comforting me?

And then I realized; she is scared, just like me. My cardiologist had mentioned this procedure several times. I didn't want to do it. One of the reasons I had been so reluctant to have the procedure is that it is technically called an EP study, short for Electro-Physiological study. The word "study" always threw me. The point of the procedure was to explore, poke around in my heart, try to replicate my extreme symptoms, then, if they could find the right places, cauterize portions of my heart. A whole new meaning to heartburn.

The kicker was that, in my particular case because of my other twenty-some symptoms, they wouldn't know if I needed the procedure until they were doing it. And they wouldn't know if they could fix my electrical conduction problem at all. Possible outcomes included: worsening of the existing condition, a Pacemaker, or death. None of those sounded worth the over $100,000 bill I would be getting as a take-home prize. Thank goodness my insurance would pay for most of it.

Despite all the risks and the ambiguity of the procedure, one thing was clear: my heart worked too hard and the intensity and frequency of the symptoms kept getting worse. All of the doctors I consulted agreed my heart couldn't handle its excessive thumping much longer.

I focused my attention back onto the bright light above me and thought about the first marathon I had ever run.

Mile marker 24, only 2.2 to go, but it was 88 degrees. Dehydrated and hallucinating, I saw rainbows and waterfalls floating in waves.

I reached out to touch them, but they disappeared, jolting me back to reality.

I had hoped to finish in under four hours, but that wouldn't happen. How had I calculated so poorly? I had chosen the Alaska marathon because I thought I'd have cool weather and nice scenery. Of course, on the date of the race there was a heat wave, the hottest recorded temperature in the history of Anchorage. The wilderness looked beautiful, but it was so hot I barely noticed. A moose, you say? Unless he had a gallon of ice cold Gatorade, I wasn't interested.

My feet pounded on the hard ground, the sun blazed down on me. There were nine miles of trails in the middle of the race without any shade. I loved running on dirt paths and rocky terrain, but there were no aid stations, and I didn't carry a water bottle because someone told me there would be no need. Aid stations every single mile, they assured me. Not so. Aid stations every two miles, and none for nine of it.

It was too late by the time I exited the narrow single track hills. The damage had been done. I tried to make up for the loss of fluids by grabbing two cups full of water as I ran past each new aid station, but it wasn't enough.

Mile 25. A tunnel. I could see it and just needed to run around the corner. I shook. Dry, salty pathways covered my arms and legs. I turned the corner and saw the final mile on a steep incline. I had been warned about it. The veterans of this race called it Heartbreak Hill.

No way. I can't do this. I'm stopping right here.

I almost stopped when I saw a boy, about five years old, standing next to what looked like his parents, cheering, smiling, and waving his hands. He made eye contact with me. His beautiful blue eyes shone bright with love. I looked straight at him, and noticed his head, bald. Bandages covered his arms.

I remembered that I wasn't running this race for me. I had raised over $3,300 to help people suffering from leukemia and lymphoma.

I had never met anyone with leukemia before. I simply wanted to help. My purple shirt, a sign of my involvement, clung to my sweaty torso, my name written across in large block letters.

The boy smiled. "Go, Cherie, you can do it!" he yelled.

Tears burst from my eyes. An uncontrollable wave of compassion almost knocked me forward. If this boy could endure chemotherapy, I could finish this last fucking mile. I would do it for him. My feet moved quicker, endorphins surged, and I ran faster than I had during the entire race.

Mile 26.2. I ran proudly across the finish line. As I took my final steps and accepted my medal, I said underneath my breath, "This is for you, little boy."

I heard a door open and shut, bringing me back into the moment. The electro-cardiologist had arrived, moving fast and fluid like a gazelle. He looked down on me and said, "Hello, Ms. Kephart." His full, pink lips matched his pink tie.

"Hi, Dr. Energized. I'm ready." I felt both scared and relieved to see him. I drew a deep breath, and from the corner of my eye I saw Dr. Eager uncap her needle.

chapter thirty

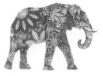

STARVING

JANUARY 2010 – LOS ANGELES

I ambled down a long concrete driveway behind my mom. I looked up into the sky and saw the L.A. smog and could almost taste it as I opened my mouth to breathe. It was familiar. It was home.

Five months since my heart surgery, I had not suffered any incidents of SVT. For this I was thankful, even though the doctor said it could come back at any time. I tried not to think about it. We believed the procedure had worked; however, the fun-filled ambiguity continued. There was no way to know what was helping: the procedure or my newest heart medication, which I needed to take until I could exercise. Exercise? My newest idea of exercise was cutting my toe nails, chewing gum, or watching HGTV (I wasn't quite ready for ESPN).

The rest of my symptoms remained unchanged, as Dr. Energized predicted. In fact, some of them had worsened. I constantly felt hungry, yet also full, a "pleasant" paradox, as if my stomach and taste buds spoke two different languages and my esophagus refused to play translator.

I continued to lose weight. My clothes hung on my frame, a reflection of a healthier time. I could no longer remember what that was like. But most importantly, my heart beat at a steady cadence. That gave me just enough ammunition to continue chasing hope.

Walking through the doorway of my great uncle Blaise's house, I soaked up my surroundings. His home looked the same as it had for decades, sixties style decor with lots of plaid and beige-colored furniture. But one thing was different. He was no longer there.

"Cherie, great to see you," my cousin Amie said, shaking me out of the daze I was in. She was petite, fit, and smelled of gardenias.

We hugged. "You too, Amie. I just wish seeing everybody was under better circumstances."

This was the first time I had been to my uncle's house since his death. I hadn't made it to his funeral since I was recovering from my heart procedure. My family understood, but I was sad, not being able to see him one last time to say goodbye.

Now, I would say goodbye, not to him, but to his house, his possessions, everything he left behind.

Amie studied me. "You look thinner than last time I saw you."

"Yeah, having trouble keeping weight on. I keep having adverse reactions to foods. All I've eaten for months is goat yogurt, brown rice, steamed vegetables, and plain baked chicken."

"Gosh, Cherie, that sounds tough."

"I call it *The No Fun Diet*."

Amie laughed. "Well, look around, and let us know if there's anything you want. We want the family to take whatever. We'll donate what's left."

I didn't want anything. I wanted my uncle back. A feisty man, with a zeal for baseball and politics, he had a way of livening up any family gathering. He was ninety-one and had lived a good life, but did that matter? There was still a hole left behind.

Six of my relatives shuffled about the house, sifting through his belongings, boxing up and stacking what needed to be hauled away.

I walked around, looking at photographs of my uncle with his buddies from the Elks lodge. He had been an active member up until his last days. I noticed exotic wooden lamps with comically carved X-rated figures, impressionistic paintings of flowers and European villages nestled by the sea, turmeric-colored lounge chairs surrounded by trinkets on shelves, and elephants. Hundreds of elephants. My aunt used to collect elephants from all over the world:

porcelain, glass, jade, stone, wooden, plastic, and even jeweled. My uncle had kept them just as she had positioned them all over the house, even though she had died several years earlier. What would become of them? Who wanted a collection of elephants? I loved elephants. And I considered taking this vast collection, but the sentimental value was lost now. These were now just items someone had once loved.

I went into the backyard. On my way out, I saw a small home-made sign sitting on the sink next to the back door in my uncle's writing. It read, "To the kind person who always brings my newspaper closer to my house, thank you. You're a thoughtful human being. I'm grateful for you."

I thought of my uncle and how difficult it had been for him to walk. He had had polio as a child, and it had returned in his old age.

The backyard was overgrown with shrubs, grass, and trees that had been neglected. Not from a lack of love, but because he was no longer there to care for them. I thought about all the times I had skirted death. What would happen to all my belongings? Did it even matter?

I ran my fingers along the jade plants, their smooth leaves comforting against my skin. I sat in the tall grass, gazing up at the one thing on my uncle's property I did want: his lemon tree. For as long as I could remember, every time I saw him, he had had a bag full of lemons. I loved lemons, particularly his. They were the juiciest ones I had ever tasted, and the lemons made me think of him.

"Cherie, you remember this old lemon tree?" my grandfather said, patting me on the back. I looked at the lemon tree, then at him, noticing his slightly crooked teeth, but at ninety-five any teeth were a gift. I studied his bulbous nose, sunken cheeks, and bald head that shined like a polished bowling ball save a few straggly white hairs.

"Yes, indeed. I love this tree." I thought about how much I loved my uncle and my grandfather. My grandfather was healthy, and for that, I was grateful. He was definitely one of my favorite people in the world.

"It sure does produce a lot of lemons. So, is there anything here you want?" He waved his arm, pointing to the garage and house. "You can have anything."

I started to say no, but then my stomach growled. "Actually Grandpa, yes, there's something I would like." I stood and half hugged him, towering over his small frame.

"Name it."

"I want some lemons."

"Lemons?" He laughed. "You don't want some paintings, jewelry, tools, furniture?"

"No, thanks. Just some lemons."

"You can have as many as you want, the tree is loaded!" He shook his head and looked toward the ground. "And golly, I know how you feel. I don't want to take anything either. I feel like a thief."

A tear leaked out from my eye. I felt frail, like death was getting closer to me. "I know, but remember, Grandpa, we aren't the thieves. Death is the thief."

chapter thirty-one

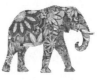

FADING

MARCH 2010 – LOS ANGELES

I am alone in a room with high ceilings and long sturdy beams. I take a deep breath, feeling the air go in, filling my lungs. I hold it, examining the beams, their width.

Alex is in the Cayman Islands for his best friend's wedding. I'm at my mother's house again in L.A. He didn't want to leave. I convinced him to go. He deserves a better life. I wonder if he will meet someone on this trip, fall in love. He could really live.

I focus back on the beams, take another deep breath.

I could swing a rope around that middle one. It would hold my weight. It would work fine. I swore I never would, but promises are sometimes tough to keep.

I exhale and gasp. Calm. There are no more tears. No more struggle. No terror. No anxiety. No desperation. Only calm.

I continue to breathe, and the air is lighter. A burden lifted. I think, no, I know, this is what has to be. There is no other choice, and I don't mind.

I write the note in my mind, line by line. The words flow easy, like sweet nectar sliding down my throat.

I think of all the parts I need to include. Everyone will want to know why. A few lines about how no one is to blame and no one should feel bad. There is no reason to. I have lived. I have loved. I am happy. I am just done. I cannot fight anymore.

I need to mention how much I love everyone, especially Alex. Because of them, I have lived a special life. Don't forget the apology. I am sorry I had to do this, but I don't view it as selfish. I need to do this so the people I love can move on with their lives and stop suffering too, since I am not the only one in pain.

I have already written my will, and Alex will take care of Ducatti. That covers everything.

I take another deep breath and reach for the rope.

chapter thirty-two

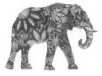

LOVE WITH LIPSTICK

MARCH 2010 – LOS ANGELES TO APRIL 2010 – SAN DIEGO

The frayed, coarse rope felt rough in my hands for three hours. I glanced away from the beams and noticed a small slice of sunlight shining across the bedroom window. Dust pirouetted in the air, and a beautiful black-and-tan butterfly floated past. The innocence of the monarch was transfixing. I saw beauty.

I then realized the magnificent beauty that had been bestowed upon me. All my friends, family, healers, doctors, and of course, Alex, who put forth such effort and love to help me survive. Gratitude filled every ounce of my being.

I let go of the rope. It dropped onto the carpet without a sound.

I would continue to fight for all the people who supported me. They deserved it. I would harness every ounce of strength and keep going. But each day was getting harder. I was so close to ending it all. How much longer could I fight?

My strength continued to plummet. I spent all my time in bed. Brenda, my therapist with the impeccable fashion sense and caring demeanor, came to my house each week and we talked. I could no longer make it to her office. She was kind enough to move our sessions to my bedside.

Alex struggled to care for me and keep up his duties at work. My grandfather kindly paid for in-home care service to come every day to make my meals, feed me, bathe me, wash my hair, clean my bedding, and do laundry—all the things I could no longer do.

Friday afternoon I sat in a wheelchair in a tiny examination room and fought to keep my eyes open as Alex and I met with my newest doctor, a rheumatologist, Dr. Genius. A serious, soft-spoken man of Russian descent, Dr. Genius had a balding head and a mustache, and always looked like a scientist studying specimens under a microscope. He was one of the brightest, most committed doctors I had ever met, and I heard from a few other patients how he had saved their lives. I hoped he could save mine.

Alex explained how fast I had deteriorated since my last appointment a short week ago and how the last few months I had rarely left my bed. Dr. Genius approached and examined my face. My stomach constricted, and my arms and feet felt numb. My head and neck felt like hundreds of tiny electric shocks were shooting through them. I started to panic, but I stifled my fear and found the strength to speak.

"I feel like I'm starving and fading, and I've started hallucinating. I can't sleep, and whenever I eat I break out in hives. I can't make it much longer like this."

"I see," he said, as if he'd already discerned that. He sat in front of me, skimmed his bare head with his hand, and sighed. "Cherie, I don't think you're going to make it through the weekend like this."

Adrenaline jolted through me. My suspicions were verified. My body was shutting down. It could take no more. I was finally dying.

Alex gripped my hand tighter. "What can we do?"

"I'll put her on steroids, to keep her going." The doctor turned to me. "You're right. You're starving; that's why you can't sleep, and why you're hallucinating. You must force yourself to eat. The steroids will help with that. And now, we wait for the test results on Monday."

Could I make it until Monday? It was the same question that had plagued me six years ago when all this started. I had suffered so much since then. I was barely alive. My answer was a powerful no.

Three hours later, the steroids ran rampant through my veins, producing artificial energy. Exhausted and manic, all my muscles felt scrawny and throbbing. My stomach distended, my heart pulsed, and my legs felt like anchors. Even my bed no longer gave me relief. It became a prison. Was this even living?

Alex yelled across the house, "They're here!"

I knew who it was, and why they were there. The muscles around my chest tightened.

Alex had called my mother while at the pharmacy and told her my status. She and my friend Jenny had both left work and driven from L.A. to be by my side to encourage me to fight, or say goodbye.

I dried my tears with a crumpled tissue, sat up in bed, and tried to gain some composure, a monumental task since my muscles strained to obey my wishes. The steroids fueled my tiny, manic movements.

"Hey, Cherie," said Jenny, a slim girl with delicate brown hair and a sincere smile.

"Hi, sweetie," said my mom, following her. "Don't worry. We're here now."

Tears pooled in the corners of my eyes. "I love you guys." I wailed.

"I love you, too," Jenny said.

"I love you, Cherie," my mom said. "And Grandpa wishes he could be here. He loves you very much."

They each held my hands. "Don't give up," Jenny said. "You've got to fight."

Please someone tell me, what am I fighting for again? I can no longer remember.

Throughout the weekend, my home bustled with activity. Alex worked. He'd been falling behind on his duties because of the time spent caring for me. My mother cleaned and cooked and Jenny ran errands.

"Alex needs me to pick up some things at the store. Is there anything else you want me to get while I'm out?" Jenny smiled. She understood I wanted love, not pity.

I shook my head, but then noticed my large bedroom mirror. "Wait. I'd like some lipstick."

"You don't wear lipstick."

"I know. Get a couple of different colors, okay?"

An hour later she returned with four different lipsticks. I took the darkest one, a shade of burgundy. Jenny helped me walk over to the mirror and propped me up against the vanity. I wrestled to stay still. My hands shook as I tried to open the shimmery silver tube. Jenny helped steady my hands. I leaned over and wrote on the mirror in front of me, "You can do this."

I handed her the lipstick. Without asking, Jenny took the lipstick, and in fancy cursive wrote, "Believe." My mom came over to see what we were doing.

I pointed to the lipsticks on the counter. "Pick a color."

My mom examined the mirror, then selected a pale pink and wrote, "You are loved."

By the end of the weekend, my large bedroom and bathroom mirrors were covered with messages in vibrant lipstick from friends, neighbors, and family who came to visit. I no longer saw my ailing reflection in the mirror. I saw a ladder.

On Monday morning, Alex held me up in the wheelchair as Dr. Genius shook my hand and sat next to me. "Cherie, how are you?"

How am I supposed to answer this? The steroids are the only thing keeping me alive.

My words came soft and slow. "Glad to still be here."

"I've got your tests. All were negative, except for one."

The word "one" hung in the air like a ghost.

"What is it?" I asked, now alert.

"Lyme."

Alex and I looked at each other, stunned. Could it be? Was it really Lyme disease all this time?

"This would explain all of your symptoms, for years, well before your collapse in 2004."

"Even her heart condition?" Alex asked.

"Yes, I believe the Lyme attacked her heart too."

"How long do you think I've had this?"

"A long time. My guess is before you went to Africa in '94."

I thought about all the unexplained symptoms I'd had over the six years, and throughout my life: neck and knee problems, a baffling and rare shoulder injury, my heart, headaches, stomach issues, depression, supposed ADHD, malaria, fibromyalgia, chronic fatigue syndrome, and the Epstein Barr. That my immune system was too feeble to fend off all those diseases in Africa made sense.

"But there's no way to know for certain," the doctor added, "and this test is inconclusive."

"What?" The obscurity of my illness, my whole life, crept back in.

"Lyme is a particularly difficult disease to test for, and prove. Your test results show that you have a ten percent chance of having Lyme, it's not for certain."

The microsecond of relief I felt disappeared.

"What do you think, doctor?" Alex asked.

"I think you have Lyme. Everything fits. These tests are not reliable, but everything you tell me makes sense. I treat the patient, not the lab tests. You've been suffering for a long time."

I felt his compassion, the spark of a fire on the winter night of this prolonged, painful illness. He believed me. I wasn't crazy. Relief flooded back. "What do we do?"

"It's a long road ahead. IV antibiotics. Very strong. Three different kinds. High doses of steroids, vitamin injections, and iron infusions since you're severely depleted. It will take many months, if not years, and won't be easy. You'll most likely get worse before you get better."

Any worse would be my cadaver being sliced open and dissected by a first-year medical student.

Dr. Genius cleared his throat. "It's called a Herxheimer reaction, or healing crisis, which is the death of bacteria or toxins in the body manifesting as severe symptoms. It's a good sign. It will show the treatments are working."

I gulped hard, figuring once again my options fell somewhere between one and none. "When do I start?"

"Tomorrow."

Three days later, Alex and my mom prepared dinner and agreed it was time for me to eat a meal at a table rather than in bed. They propped me up in my chair, where I stared at a plate of chicken, rice, and steamed vegetables. I had no strength to lift a glass. My mom bought plastic cups and straws so I could drink unassisted.

I tried to harness the strength to pick up my fork and take a bite of chicken, but I had trouble focusing. Little opaque spots formed in front of my eyes and unforgiving pangs pulsed inside me. A thunderstorm of shrapnel exploded inside my neck, back, shoulders, and chest every time I inhaled.

I hallucinated again, watching thick dark clouds fill our dining room. Black rain poured over me, each raindrop feeling as if a scalpel sliced open my flesh. Blood ran down my arms and legs and dripped onto the stone floor. My face flushed, my muscles tightened, and the room spun. I flinched and gasped. *What's happening?*

Alex and my mom ate their meals, unaware of my furrowed brow and the drop of my head toward my lap. They seemed miles away, in another galaxy, while I slipped in and out of consciousness.

I lifted my right hand from my thigh up toward the table, resting it next to my plate beside the serrated edge of my knife. I imagined picking it up and plunging it deep inside my heart, twisting it until I stopped breathing.

I took a deliberate breath, clutched the knife, and lifted it toward my chest. I brought the knife in closer. It would all be over soon.

The cold, sharp tip of the knife touched my skin. I gripped the knife tighter, then I heard a voice. *Cherie, no!*

My voice. The resilient woman imprisoned inside this insanity. Still in there somewhere. *Don't do it. Throw the knife down, now!*

I released the knife and started to sob. I screamed, "Help!"

Alex jumped up from his seat. "What's wrong?"

"Please! Take the knife away."

"Wha…"

My hands shook. I motioned to the knife. "Please. I almost plunged it into my chest."

Alex grabbed the knife and put it at the other end of the table. My mom and Alex rushed to my side and cradled me. I collapsed in their arms.

"I don't want to die," I wailed, tears streaming down my chin.

"We know. We're here, Cherie. We're not leaving you," they said, their voices overlapping.

Out of the corner of my eye, I could see the knife at the other end of the table, shimmering in the glow of the chandelier, beckoning me.

Then a figure appeared near the knife. It was the little boy from the marathon, the one with leukemia. A white glow outlining his body. A white baseball cap covered his bald head. The inscription on his cap read, "Be My Hero."

chapter thirty-three

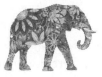

So Much More

OCTOBER 2010 – SAN DIEGO

After almost six months of exhausting IV treatments, about four hours each day, five days a week, and swallowing forty-six pills a day, I felt a shift, like a wave of peace slowly moving through me, healing my body, mind, and soul. The twenty-seven different symptoms I had had since 2004 were at least cut in half. I was finally on the path! I was healing! I ate unassisted, even prepared a few meals. The day I put my shower chair in the attic was euphoric. Perhaps one day I could be completely healthy.

The week before my sixth and final month of IV treatments, I had one of the worst pains ever. It felt like a rhinoceros was sitting on my chest, while a boulder the size of Canada tried to push itself through a space inside me meant for the passage of a sunflower seed.

The large quantity and types of drugs I had taken had caused my liver enzymes to skyrocket, and gallstones had formed. One of them tried to pass through where it could never fit. I was alone, so I called 911. I remember thinking: *If I had a gun, I would shoot myself.*

When the paramedics came to my house for the umpteenth time, they told me to calm down. I thought: *Give me pain meds NOW or I'll shoot you too.*

They took me to the hospital without any meds.

After I was admitted to my own room at the hospital, a heavy dose of pain medications filtered through my veins, finally soothing me. I flipped through a medical magazine and found an article about Lyme disease. The first line was all I needed.

Cherie Kephart

"Lyme disease is one of the most controversial illnesses in the history of medicine."

A hospital physician, Dr. Grim, told me I had to stay in the hospital until my liver enzymes dropped back to a normal range in the 20s. When I arrived, they were over 1,100. I could have died from liver failure from the treatments trying to save me.

Or a gunshot.

A few weeks after my release from the hospital, I met with Dr. Genius. He entered the exam room with a stack of lab tests in his hands. "Cherie, I believe the treatments have worked. There's no certainty, but the Lyme may be in remission."

I cried, but this time, they were happy tears. "Oh my God! Thank you so much, doctor."

Alex held me close. Out of the corner of my eye I could see him wiping tears from his eyes.

Dr. Genius nodded and flashed a modest smile. "It's not over. Now, we need to focus on repairing the long-term damage and treat the many other ailments. Your body's been through a lot. This will take some time, most likely years. We also need to treat you for post-traumatic stress disorder. This will play a huge factor in your recovery. But I'm confident." He shook my hand, then Alex's hand, and left.

I wasn't the only one with PTSD. Alex suffered from it too. He felt on edge every day, wondering when would be the next time I would call his name, screaming and pleading to be taken back to the hospital. Each day that I wasn't being tortured was also a day when Alex was given back a little bit of his life.

I turned to Alex and grinned. "We did it! I'm starting to heal!"

"You did it, CK. I can't even imagine how difficult it's been for you."

"And I can't imagine how hard it's been for you. Thank you, Alex. You're wonderful!"

He hugged me and whispered in my ear, "I know."

224

chapter thirty-four

BURN TO LIVE

FEBRUARY 2011 – SAN DIEGO

After months of physical, neurological, and emotional therapy, I felt stronger. I walked up to five minutes each day, wrote, read, and even started driving short distances. Although I still had several symptoms and was still unsure if Lyme disease was my true diagnosis, I was on an upward trajectory. I felt like a turtle heading for a piece of lettuce, slow, yet nevertheless determined.

I realized there wasn't one thing in particular that helped me begin to heal; it was a hundred. The treatments, the heart procedure, meditation, affirmations, caring physicians, healers, nurses, my supportive family and friends, my newfound peace and appreciation for living in the moment, truly letting go, accepting accountability for my choices and everything that had led me here, and finally, my belief in something bigger in this universe than my tiny life. It was transformative and took years. And it was just the beginning.

My doctors all agreed it was time for me to get out and be social, that it would help my healing. They often asked me, "What do you do for fun?"

I couldn't answer. I hadn't thought about fun for years. I'd been trying not to die! I figured I would have fun again when I was well. How silly of me to not realize having some fun would help me heal.

After much deliberation and searching for some sort of activity that I could do, I joined a poetry group at the local senior center. With my Medicare card, emergency contact information, hefty supply of Benadryl, heart medication, no-frills supportive walking shoes, and handicap placard, I fit right in. My thirty-nine-year-old body felt like ninety-three, and was living like it too. I wondered, where had all the years gone? Next stop, Bingo.

It felt invigorating to be out in the world, to be on my own, not in a doctor's office. I felt a glimmer of freedom. It felt wonderful.

While sitting on the couch working on my latest poem, I stroked Ducatti's silky black fur. I felt warmth in my heart as I heard him purr. Twelve years as my companion, and he still gave me such love. I leaned over and gave him a big kiss. He didn't even open his eyes; he merely stretched and moved into a tighter upside down head tuck. He scored ten out of ten on the cuteness scale.

I reread the last few lines of my poem, and a hollow sensation filled my lungs.

> *...And I walk small through the forest*
> *of dark thoughts asking to be shown*
> *the path, yet it is only when I stand*
> *tall that I make my own way*
> *to the place illuminated by peace.*

I closed my journal and headed upstairs to Alex's office. He looked up from his laptop. "You ready?"

I smiled. "Yes."

An hour later Alex drove me down to the fire pits at Moonlight Beach. "I'll be in the car if you need me."

"Thank you, Alex. For everything. You're the best!" I flung my arms around him.

"I know." He laughed and hugged me back.

I could feel the love in his embrace. It resembled a sunrise, the beauty and promise of a new day. We were like war buddies, having endured something that no one else could understand. We didn't know what the future would hold for us, but we did know we would always be close.

I got out of the car and headed toward the sand. I squatted in front of a fire pit with four large paper bags full of stuff, newspaper, and a couple of thin pieces of kindling. It was a serendipitous location to conduct a burning ritual, since this was where I used to play beach volleyball in my healthier times. Perhaps a sign of the future, I hoped.

Amongst a beach full of people, I sat alone on the sand with a box of matches and my four large piles of fuel. With my iPod playing some of the most soulful and inspiring music I could think of, the perfect piano of Fabrizio Paterlini, I made a bonfire and watched item by item go up in flames. Lyme disease lab tests, heart procedure bills, thousands of heart-rate monitoring printouts and EKGs, car-accident paperwork, police paperwork, medical bills, disability papers, a skirt I had worn when I spoke at Bruce's funeral, and several other artifacts representing a variety of times that I was ready to release.

I thought about many other doctors I had seen as I held a crumpled list of all their names in my hand: Dr. Agreeable, Dr. Arrogant, Dr. Awkward, Dr. Blank-Stare, Dr. Cookie-Cutter, Dr. Curt, Dr. Cynical, Dr. Gorilla-Hands, Dr. Guy-I-Used-To-Date, Dr. Handsome, Dr. Hormone, Dr. Jovial, Dr. Nervous, Dr. Pricey, Dr. Psychic, Dr. Rescue, Dr. Serious, Dr. Stand-up Comedian, Dr. Trauma, Dr. Wacky, and Dr. Zoologically Inclined, then threw it into the fire.

I also made a list of all the things I wanted for the future and burned that too, with the idea that, by releasing them into the world, they would come true.

The smell of the smoke reminded me of Zambia with all the fires in my village and hundreds of people cooking their millet and dried fish in the ground outside their mud huts. I fondly remembered my time there, and felt happiness for the adventures I had survived. I wondered about Fewdays. I wrote to him several times after I returned to the states, but only heard from him once, then never again. I hoped one day to find him.

After almost two hours of placing item after item in the fire, spreading the ashes, and ensuring everything stayed in the pit, I felt hot and tired, but I was finished and felt free. I stood up, watched the last flames extinguish and morph into gray ash, turned away, and without looking back, walked down a short trail to the ocean.

I passed a crushed snail on the pavement. Next to it stood a trash can full of ants feasting on the remnants of a partially eaten chicken breast. Two women walked their dogs, conversing about a relative who had passed away. On a grassy knoll, a bird slurped up a freshly plucked worm from the ground, and the remains of a squirrel lay sprawled next to the edge of the sidewalk, the victim of a vehicular accident. Death was everywhere. Why did I think I could avoid it?

I arrived at the end of the pathway, kicked off my flip flops, and sat cross-legged on the sand, pushing it through my toes and arching my back and head up to the heat of the sun.

I gazed out onto the shimmering water. The waves swept in and out before me, hypnotizing my senses, and silencing my fears.

A flock of tiny brown and white birds flew down onto the wet sand in front of me and ran toward the frothy waves, poking their heads into the sodden sand, searching for food. As the water rushed forward, they scattered back to the beach.

I watched them hunt for nourishment. I noticed one bird hopping along with only one functional leg. Despite his hardship, he leapt forward and kept up with the others. He had no choice but to stay tough. After watching him hobble and scurry along, I thought of how I had relied on countless factors to survive my illness. This little bird relied only on himself.

And then, in the reflection of the water, the little boy from the marathon appeared. His bright eyes shone, his arms waving hello to me.

My heart burst with love. I waved back to him and I mouthed, "Thank you."

He grinned with delight, and as fast as he appeared, he floated up and faded away into the golden rays of the sun that peeked through the clouds.

Minutes later, I climbed back up the small hill. My breathing was labored. I stopped halfway to catch my breath and saw a woman pushing a stroller with twin babies snuggled in fuzzy blankets, sleeping peacefully. Two crows flew above me, squawking and swooping alongside each other. A pregnant woman sat on a bench sipping coffee, watching her toddler play on a nearby swing set. Close to the car, a teenage couple held hands and gazed at each other as if they were the only two souls on the earth. Goose bumps prickled my forearms.

Death was everywhere, but so was life.

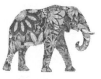

ACKNOWLEDGMENTS

How many people does it take to help an author write her book? How many people does it take to save this author's life?

The answer: a lot.

This book is my way of saying thank you to everyone who supported me, both in writing this book and in saving my life. The list is long, and of that, I am proud and full of gratitude.

I am grateful to my editors. To Mark Clements: Thank you for believing in me from the very beginning (did I just use the word *very?*—egad!), and for sharing your most valuable time and expertise. Indeed, your willingness to mentor me and so many other writers is a gift to this craft. To Marni Freedman: My spiritual sister and structure queen, you are so talented. I'm forever fortunate to have met you. Thank you for enhancing my book and my life. To Peggy Lang: Thank you for your ongoing encouragement, sound advice, and thoughtfulness throughout this whole journey. You are an example of true generosity and coaching with heart. To Matthew J. Pallamary: I am grateful for your keen eye, mindful suggestions, and exceptional mentoring. With you by my side, I have blossomed as a writer. You are confirmation that spirit matters. To Alex Sheshunoff: What a joy to meet someone so open and devoted to writers and writing. Thank you for your counsel, your humor, and for paying it forward. To all of you: I will continue to do for others what you have done for me.

To Asa Wild: Thank you for your stunning cover and interior design, and your constancy in all facets of this book and in my life.

Your friendship is a beacon of light, keeping me on the path. I can only hope I can be as valuable to you as you have been to me.

To my writing group, my mentors, and all my fellow writers, your continued encouragement, constructive advice, and stamina through this lengthy book writing process has been both an anchor and a kite—keeping me grounded while helping me fly. Special thanks to Anna-Marie Abell, Susan Banks, Roger Conlee, Carla King, Paul De Lancey, Norm DeWitt, Diane Dettman, Anastasia Hipkins, Clifton King, Reina Mensache, Eliza Rhodes, Lindsey Salatka, Gerardeen Santiago, Jeff Thurman, Barbara Villaseñor, Karl Weiss, and Dilia Wood. You have elevated this book and my experience as a writer. I feel honored to be a part of such an awesome writing family.

To all my doctors, nurses, healers, therapists, medical assistants, and everyone in the medical community, especially those at the Institute for Specialized Medicine and Scripps Hospitals and Clinics: Thank you for all you have done for me and so many others with difficult-to-diagnose illnesses. I do not remember or even know the names of all the hundreds, maybe thousands of people that have helped me along this healing journey. I do know that I would not be alive without your knowledge, devotion, and compassion. Special thanks to: Dr. Andrew Blumenfeld, Dr. Martin Charlat, Dr. Thomas Fay, Dr. Ali Hamzei, Dr. Dan Harper, Dr. Michael Haug, Dr. Karen Lee, Dr. Warren Levin, Dr. Benjo Masilungun, Dr. Melinda Nevins, Dr. Lisa Petri, Dr. Alexander Shikhman, Dr. Anne Smith, Dr. Raymond Woo, Dr. Mario Yco, Tenia Bentley, Master John Douglas, Erika Gleva, Beverly Hamowitz, Steve Hansen, Satya and Michael Hurley, Tom and Trisha Kelly, Diane and Randy Kusuhose, Kathleen Larson, David Lemberg, Willow MacPherson, Shelley McQuerter, Paula Milford, Vicki Murphy, Brigitte Noel, Marsha Norris, Debbie Novick, Flossie Park, Suresh Ramaswamy, Christina Sandoval, MJ Schwader, Crespina Senteno, and Linda Smith. You are truly saviors. I am forever grateful and humbled by your devotion to helping people heal. Always know that I am healing and living a truly incredible life because you took the time to care. I will never forget.

To my fellow Zambia Peace Corps volunteers, the *Kalapashi*: *Natotela sana mukwai*, for being my family away from family: Kala Bokelman, Roy Brennen, Counsella Brown, Roslyn Docktor, Joe Ford, Andy and Renate Girard, Chris and Helen Haydon, Greg Irish, Daniel Kuhn, Peter Meerbergen, Michelle Milne, Sarina Ochoa, Ken Puvak, and Josh Swiller. You are a testament to all the good in the world. No matter the time or space between us, I will carry you with me in all my adventures. Also, to the incredible Susan Ackerman, who is partially to blame for my time in Zambia. Thank you for this invaluable gift through which I have learned to see the truth in the world and in myself.

To all the wonderful people in Zambia who accepted this light-haired, blue-eyed, left-handed, sports-bra wearing, completely-out-of-place California girl who invaded your country with her childlike dreams and landed back home with grace in her heart from all you gave to her: *Cibote*.

To Fewdays Chipili: May you know I will always look for you in the glow of the stars and in every cliché ever written. My appreciation for your friendship will travel for eternity.

To Bruce Wilson: I still haven't been able to ride a bike. Looks like I'm saving it for when I see you again. Thank you, my friend, for all the love. One day we will ride free.

To my many beautiful friends: What can a girl say except I am alive because of you. I am alive for you. I am here for you. Thank you for making my life extraordinary. I especially want to thank the remarkable: Carol Bourgoin, Anthony Breunig, Anton, Sheila, and Maria Calleia, Ron Cole, Alex Dee, Jean Demeo, Jurgen Dentener, Mike Ewer, CJ Frey, Maximillian Gasseholm, Steven Gregory, Kevin Grold, Peter Hammonds, Paul Johnson, Mike and Nancy Kauffman, Joe King, Chris and Marsha Kitzmiller, Mark and Teresa Lloyd, Nicole Martel, Joyce and Laura Matlack, Peg Miller, Catey Moore, Shirley Munch, Brigid Parsons, Julie Poehnelt, Rob Reed, Jonathan Reinstein, Stacie Bresler-Reinstein, Dennie Shypryt-Knoop, Andrew Simpson, Cibele Sousa, Robert and Olga Stebbins, Jean Steinemann,

Sharon Sternfeld, Matthew Taylor, Saurabh Thaper, Peter Van Kemseke, Debra Wanger, Regina Wilson, Sara Wingate, and Hillary Vari. You stood by me all this time, stepped in and helped me when I needed you most. You cared for me while my body, mind, and spirit felt shattered, and lifted me up above the clouds to face the sun. My infinite love and gratitude is yours.

To Priscilla Gale: From our days in junior high drinking dill pickle juice and sporting horrific 1980s hairstyles to college, difficult relationships, and our painful health challenges; our bond is unbreakable. No matter the physical miles between us, you are with me in each moment. Thank you especially for accepting me for exactly who I am, never judging, always loving.

Thank you to my family. My mom, Linda: Thank you for always being there when I truly needed you. May you have peace in your heart knowing that your daughter is proud to call you mother. To my dad, Arthur: Thank you for teaching me to follow my unique life's path and for always knowing when to listen and let me be me. To my brother, Tom: Thank you for mentoring me, being patient as I navigated making mistakes, and most of all for agreeing to never play Monopoly with me ever again. To my beautiful big sister, Lisa: Thank you for your undeniable bigheartedness and generosity. You helped me be strong and, without prompting, gave when I needed it the most. To my sister-in-law, Lori: Thank you for your compassion, dedication to our family, and for raising the loveliest three kids. To my brother-in-law, Jonathan: Thank you for being the best xylophone soloist ever known and for bringing even more love and happiness to my sister's life.

Thanks to my niece, Katie, for her grace and courage, and to my nephews, Bob and Joe, for their humor and magnificent presence that is a delight to be around. To my aunts, uncles, and cousins, for being there for me no matter how much time passes. To my cousin Matt: Thanks for lifting me up, keeping me laughing, and being there during my darkest times. To Cameron and Caitlin: Thank you for your acceptance and love; you have made my life richer.

To all my family who have passed on, you will always be with me. To my grandmother, Lucile: Thank you for your caring ways and infectious laughter; I miss you. To my grandfather, Joseph, who recently died at one-hundred-years-old: Thank you for the most unconditional love I have ever felt.

To Brian Eslick: My everlasting gratitude to you for being such a pristine source of friendship, laughter, encouragement, and of course, maximum-strength love. Your positivity and devoutness has been paramount to my healing. You are a miraculous man, and I am honored to know and love you.

To all my adorable furry feline children, all of whom are in kitty heaven drinking tuna juice and lounging in the bright light of the sun: Thank you for your years of comfort and companionship. I never felt alone with you by my side, especially around feeding time.

My most endearing gratitude goes to my adoring feline Ducatti—thank you for seventeen years of pure love. Not only are you still my longest male relationship, but you will always be the coolest guy in any room. I love and miss you and look forward to one day being with you again.

To all those who suffer from chronic illnesses, diagnosed or undiagnosed: Your ongoing strength and will to live inspire me. To my dearest friends: Ivy Aubry, Jennifer Dunn, Amanda Duty, Michelle Goodsell, Jannet McCuthchen, Azadeh Montaser, Beth Nelson, Jo Rabin, Marshall Ross, Cathie Smith, and Kika Sales, thank you for sharing this journey with me and for never giving up.

To Christine Hartline-Grold: I know you are at peace now. I miss you always and know that our friendship transcends all time and space, even beyond life. I am making each day count.

Lastly, to Alex: I can never write anything for you, to you, or about you without crying. This is no exception. Just know whatever you need, wherever you are, I am there for you. Your unwavering support and love gave me a second chance. For this, and everything you have done for me, I am grateful evermore.

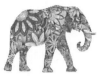

ABOUT THE AUTHOR

Raised in Venice, California, Cherie longed to travel and experience the way other people lived. After serving as a Peace Corps volunteer in Zambia on a water sanitation and health education project, Cherie returned to the United States with an African souvenir she didn't expect: a mysterious illness. She fell severely ill and almost died, leaving her with symptoms that went undiagnosed for many years. This inspired Cherie to write her memoir, *A Few Minor Adjustments: A Memoir of Healing*, taking the reader on a powerful-but-entertaining journey through her adventures and search for life-saving answers.

A graduate of the University of Auckland, New Zealand with an M.A. in Medical and Cultural Anthropology with First Class Honors, Cherie also holds a B.A. in Communications from UCSD and a Certification in Scientific and Technical Writing.

A Few Minor Adjustments is a 2017 San Diego Book Awards winner. It was also featured in the San Diego Memoir Showcase and was performed onstage at the Horton Grand Theater. Cherie's essays, stories, and poems have appeared in publications and events such as: *The San Diego Poetry Annual*, *The San Diego Writers Ink Anthology*, Oceanside Literary Art Walk, Wild Lemon Project, *Magee Park Poets Anthology*, and in the Transform Your Life classes.

After traveling to more than forty countries, Cherie now lives in San Diego and is passionate about healing the body, mind, and spirit, and sharing her experiences to help others. She has been celebrated for her holistic approach to healing, and her willingness to examine her life lessons in her writing.

Look for her future publications and stay connected with Cherie at: CherieKephart.com

Stay Involved

Connect with Cherie on her Website

CherieKephart.com

Write a Review

for *A Few Minor Adjustments*
CherieKephart.com/review

Connect with Cherie on Social Media

@Cherie.Kephart.Author

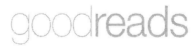

Cherie Kephart

@CherieKephart

CPSIA information can be obtained
at www.ICGtesting.com
Printed in the USA
FSOW01n1530270917
38816FS

9 781947 127012